Kolinka Zinovieff qualified as an Aromatherapist at the Institute of Clinical Aromatherapy and studied a postgraduate course at L'Institute des Sciences Phytomédicales. He also trained as a Craniosacral Therapist with the CrOA (Cranial Osteopathic Association) and at the Upledger Institute. He is on the inner council of the BCMA (British Complementary Medicine Association). Kolinka can be contacted at 10 Bamborough Gardens, London, W12 8QN (telephone (44) 0181 743 9485).

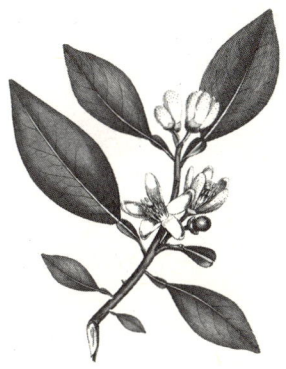

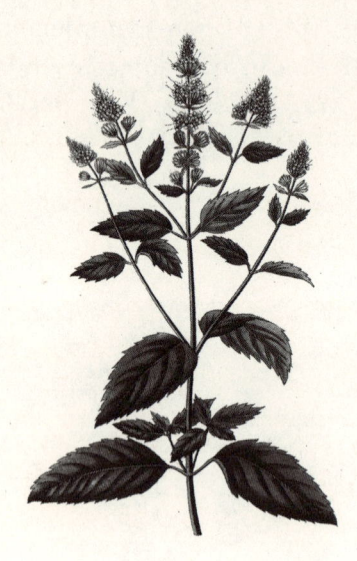

Natural Aromatherapy Remedies

The Complete Home Guide

By

Kolinka Zinovieff

Natural Aromatherapy Remedies

The Complete Home Guide

By Kolinka Zinovieff

Published
by
London Natural Health Press
10 Bamborough Gardens
London W12 8QN

ISBN 0-9527825-0-2

Copyright © 1996 Kolinka Zinovieff

Printed in Great Britain

Important note

The information in this book is not intended as a replacement for medical advice. Any person with a medical or health problem should consult a qualified health care professional. Aromatherapy is not a replacement for orthodox medicine, it can support the treatment your doctor is giving you.

PERSONAL INTRODUCTION

My own experience of illness lasted for four years. It showed me that illness can enrich our lives and help us learn life's lessons in a more fulfilling way. I would not deny the great pain and difficulty involved, but would simply emphasise that illness can, if we allow it, be an opportunity to change our lives for the better.

For me, being ill for that time gave me an opportunity to put aside all the old habits and ways: a chance to start life afresh. I began to feel a new sense of an inner respect which involved honouring the body's need to be ill while at the same time looking at the root causes for the condition.

Sometimes illnesses have obvious causes which may be of an emotional, mental, environmental or energetic kind. At other times they can be a lesson in letting go of the mind and accepting the body's need to be ill. There does not seem to be any easy solution but our attitude toward illness can make all the difference. Our view of illness as an enemy that needs to be suppressed and got rid of at all costs, may change to one where we perceive it as a friend. Then we can begin to feel it is offering us an opportunity to learn about ourselves and a chance to make our experience of life richer and more rewarding.

Aromatherapy is one way in which we can begin this process of healing and nourishing ourselves at all levels: physical, emotional, mental and spiritual. I hope you find this book of use and enjoy using nature's healing essential oils.

ACKNOWLEDGEMENTS

Firstly, I would like to thank our Mother earth for providing us with these noruishing oils which are helping so many people, as well as giving me the pleasure of writing about them.

I would especially like to thank - Ben Ellis for his support and suggestions and proof reading, Renáta Tichá for her highly skilled proof reading, Rand Marsh for his contributions and my father Peter Zinovieff for his beautiful layout and editing. I would also like to thank Zofia and Tim Hockin, and Nicky O'Hara.

Lastly, I thank my dog Billy who patiently waited for me and encouraged me to go for walks.

A blank page for your notes

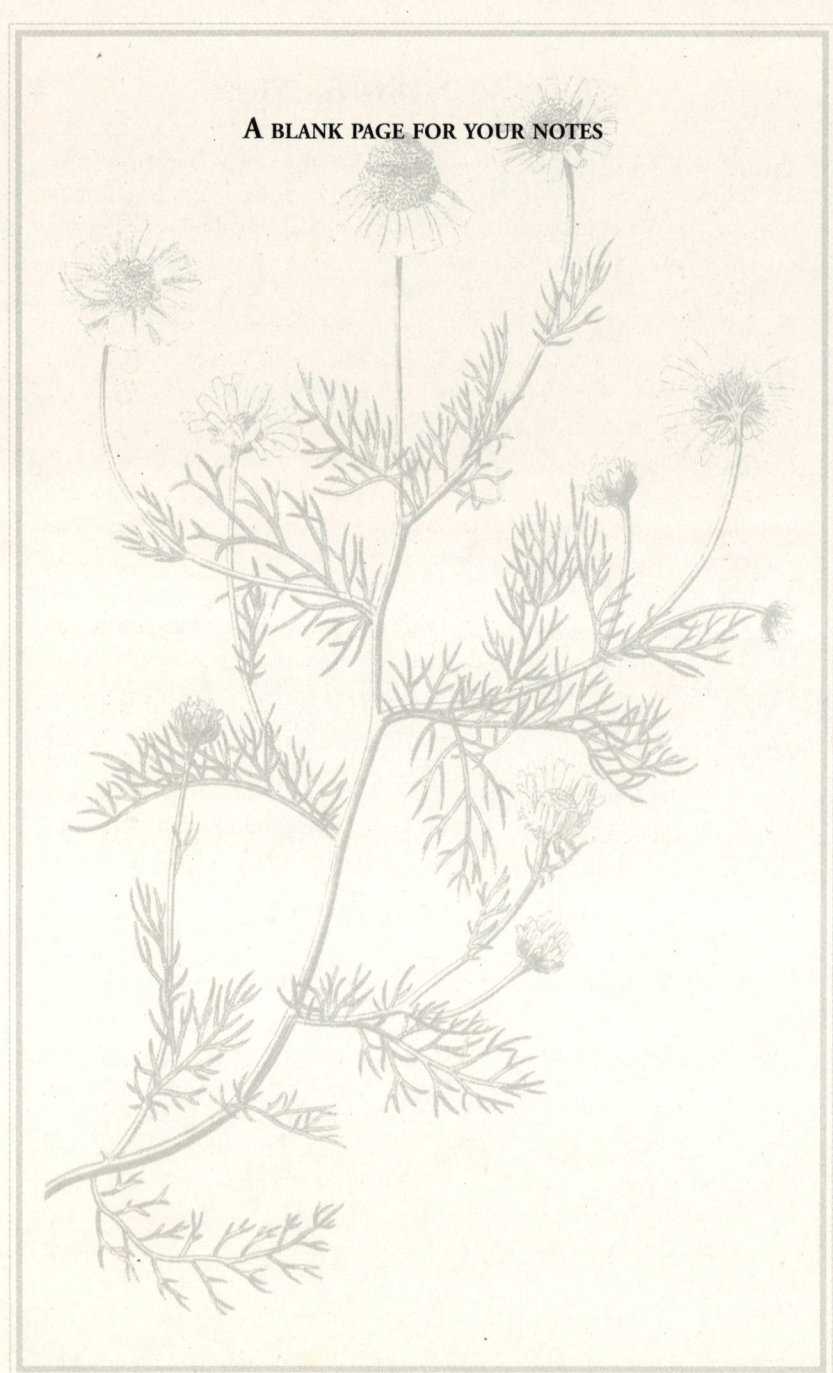

CONTENTS

	Page
PERSONAL INTRODUCTION	5
ACKNOWLEDGEMENTS	5
INTRODUCTION	8
HISTORY OF AROMATHERAPY	9
HOW ESSENTIAL OILS ARE OBTAINED	11
HOW ESSENTIAL OILS WORK	14
HOW TO USE ESSENTIAL OILS AT HOME	16
WARNINGS	19
AN A-Z OF COMMON AILMENTS	20
THE ESSENTIAL OILS	43
CASE HISTORIES	54
MEDITATION	59
RECOMMENDED FURTHER READING	60
USEFUL ORGANISATIONS	61
GLOSSARY	63

INTRODUCTION

Natural remedies are enjoying a great revival and especially in the use of essential oils and herbal medicine. This is partly due to an increasing sense of disillusionment with orthodox medicine and partly to a new awareness of the successful alternatives in use by other peoples all over the world.

Although we should not ignore the great benefits medical science has and is giving us, the present trend of treating conditions and illnesses with powerful modern chemical drugs with little regard to the emotional, psychological and environmental background of each case and each individual, is proving dangerously short-sighted. The use of such drugs for almost any ailment, causes serious side-effects and a possible slow breakdown of the body's immune system. In contrast, natural medicines (such as Aromatherapy) help the body's own immune system to function more efficiently on a holistic level without unwanted side-effects or addictive tendencies. That said, it is important for both types of medicine to work in partnership, sharing the best qualities in each area. I look forward to this time which is already starting now.

Industrial and scientific advancement in the West saw an evolution towards man-made medicines and drugs and a decline in our knowledge and respect for natural medicines. Simultaneously there developed the loss of respect for nature and our environment. Today we are witnessing a global reawakening in the awareness of the consequences of our destructive actions against our Mother, the earth. We must take care to conserve the world's potential. For instance, the continuing tragic loss of our rainforests causes the inevitable extinction of healing herbs and plants. We simply do not have any idea of what we might be losing.

There is an increasing number of people taking responsibility for their own health care. In fact, the fastest growing area of medicine is what is often labelled "alternative medicine" or, to be more precise, "complementary" medicine which is a clearer name for working in cooperation with or complementing orthodox medicine. In acute conditions, where modern techniques, such as surgery, are needed, orthodox medicine is far more appropriate. Yet, even here, Aromatherapy can be used to help in the recovery from these treatments. In areas of preventative medicine and in the treatment of common ailments, such as colds, flus and long term conditions where orthodox medicine offers no treatments, complementary medicine (e.g. Aromatherapy) is often much more effective. It is important to have a balanced respect for both systems and the knowledge to use each appropriately.

On a personal note, I feel a great gratitude towards nature for these precious essential oils. They have helped me recover from a long and difficult illness and they continue to help me balance and harmonise my life. I never go far without my kit of oils for all eventualities: Lavender, Tea-Tree, Geranium and Frankincense are my trusted friends.

HISTORY OF AROMATHERAPY

Essential oils and aromatic plants have been used for healing purposes over thousands of years by all the great civilisations of the world, such as the Greek, Roman, Egyptian, Chinese and Indian.

In 2000 BC an ancient Vedic text of India reports over 700 herbs and oils in use for healing. Egyptian sources dating back as far as 2800 BC (1st and 2nd Dynasties) record the use of many medicinal herbs for healing, aromatic substances for embalming process and the scents of aromatic oils, such as Eucalyptus, Lavender, and Clove, were used to treat skin disorders. In many ancient societies herbs and oils were often so valuable and highly sought after that they were even used as currency.

Hypocrites, often called the 'Father of Medicine', recommended aromatic baths and scented massage to enhance health and prolong life.

There is an ever expanding growth in the present-day use of Aromatherapy as a healing technique. This resurgence was spearheaded by the French chemist René Maurice Gattefosse who, in 1930, discovered that essential oils used for cosmetic purposes also had medicinal applications. One day, while working in his laboratory, Dr. Gattefosse badly burned his hand and accidentally put it into Lavender oil, the closest liquid in reach. He was amazed how soothing the Lavender oil felt, and how quickly the burn healed, leaving no scar. This accident sparked his interest in researching the healing properties of essential oils. Dr. Gattefosse successfully treated many wounded soldiers using essential oils. It was he who first coined the word 'Aromatherapie' to describe healing treatments using essential oil: 'aroma' for the importance of smell and 'therapie' to describe the effect of healing.

This century has seen a continuous progress in the scientific research into the effects of essential oils used in Aromatherapy. Today, even in 'orthodox medicine' essential oils are used in prescriptions and over the counter medicines. Doctors now prescribe throat lozenges and tablets which contain Tea-Tree oil (these can be bought from chemists). In Australia various antiseptics in hospitals now include Tea Tree oil because of its effective antibacterial and antiviral properties. In France many doctors are also Aromatherapists and routinely prescribe essential oils for ailments instead of chemical drugs. Many pharmaceutical ointments and antiseptics contain Lavender and Tea-Tree as well as other essential oils.

The consumer industry uses essential oils in detergents, soaps, cosmetics, perfumes and in flavouring. Peppermint oil is widely used in chewing gums, alcoholic drinks, toothpaste and as flavouring in various foods and remedies. Lemon is used in a huge variety of drinks and foods.

Some historical facts

▶▶ Aromatic substances were one of the earliest world trade items, being rare and highly valuable.

▶▶ The earliest texts on Aromatherapy are from ancient Egypt, during the reign of Khufu, and are dated 2800 BC

▶▶ In the Bible the Book of Exodus describes that the Lord transmitted to Moses a formula for a special anointing oil which included the essential oils Myrrh and Cinnamon.

▶▶ Frankincense and myrrh (from which essential oils can be made) were great treasures of the East. They were offered to Jesus at his birth.

▶▶ Tutankhamun's tomb still had traces and odour of aromatic oils when opened in 1922.

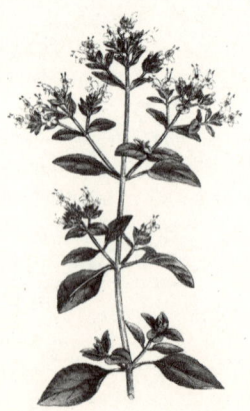

HOW ESSENTIAL OILS ARE OBTAINED

How wonderful are some of the memories that are triggered by a smell: the burst of the essence of a tangerine from a Christmas stocking, a walk through a rose garden on a summer afternoon, fresh pine needles while hiking in the woods, lavender or rosemary picked in a vegetable garden or wild thyme spotted on a Scottish moor and rubbed between the fingers.

These familiar fragrances, which we know and love, come from the actual essential oils of these same plants. Some parts of plants, like the peel of an orange, contain large quantities of oil, others, such as rose petals, contain tiny amounts. The oily substance seen and smelt when peeling an orange is the essential oil itself oozing out, making it very easy to extract and hence one of the least expensive oils. Rose oil, on the other hand, is extremely expensive because it takes one ton of rose petals to produce 1 pint of essential oil.

EXTRACTION

'**Steam Distillation**' is the most common way to obtain essential oils. The plant material (for example, lavender) is placed in water which is boiled, the mixture coming off is then cooled and condenses into water and essential oil. The essential oil is collected and the water is either thrown away or used as a floral water.

'**Expression**' is the simplest method of extraction and is applied mainly to citrus fruits (e.g. orange, lemon). The rinds of the fruits are compressed or grated to force out the oil. Centrifuges are often used to assist the process.

'**Solvent Extraction**' is the usual method used to extract floral oils (e.g. Jasmine, Rose) where the plants yield very small amounts of oil. The flowers are covered in a solvent (for example hexane or petroleum ether) which dissolves the oil. The solvent is then either evaporated or distilled away, leaving behind the pure oil. Oil produced in this way is very concentrated and is called 'absolute' to distinguish it from 'normal' oil made by other methods. Huge amounts of flowers are needed to produce tiny quantities of absolute oil. Hence the great expense of oils such as Rose, Jasmine and Neroli.

SYNERGISTIC BLENDS

Synergistic blends are created when two or more essential oils are mixed together to make a dynamic combination or blend, which is more powerful than the unblended individual oils. The whole becomes greater than the sum of the parts. Certain essential oils complement each other when mixed together. It is important to use the right combination of oils to create this synergy; for example, when Lavender and Camomile are combined the anti-inflammatory actions of the Camomile are greatly increased.

In the 'A-Z of Common Complaints' section, the essential oils which have an asterisk against them create particularly powerful synergistic blends.

QUALITY

Because it can be so costly to produce Aromatherapy essential oils, there is a great temptation for manufacturers to dilute the oils or use cheaper man-made chemical ingredients. Such chemical adulterations or synthetic oils have **no** therapeutic or healing qualities whatsoever: indeed, the oils may actually be harmful. If you discover very cheap essential oils, you can be guaranteed that they are not pure and natural. Great care and discrimination should be used when buying oils. The best method is to see what the average price is in different shops and avoid any oils that are much lower in price. You almost always pay for the quality you get.

Many perfumes and oils originally obtained from flowers (e.g. lilac and carnation) are nowadays almost entirely synthetically produced. Such synthetic oils are called 'nature identical' and are used by the perfume and food industries which need large quantities of cheap and readily available oils. To make a cheap synthetic oil, one or two of the main aromatic ingredients of the natural oil are synthetically copied and mass produced. Natural oils themselves are always highly complex substances and contain hundreds of individual ingredients often in minuscule proportions. It is impossible to make a perfect copy of them.

The therapeutic power of natural oils is due, in part, to their complexity. The different ingredients have a synergistic effect with each other. This is the wonderful mystery which continues to baffle the over-rational scientific mind. We are still a long way from being able to copy, let alone fully understand, the complexity of these beautiful oils that nature has given us.

The other area of quality one needs to pay attention to when buying oils is to know which are organic or wild grown (that is from plants cultivated without the use of pesticides or chemicals). Organically grown oils are much more potent and pure, thus enhancing their therapeutic and healing effects. Chemicals and fertilisers used in non-organic farming are often absorbed into the plant and hence into the body when using non-organic oils, thereby reducing their healing properties.

The quality of essential oils is affected by two main factors:

First, the quality of the original plant, i.e. whether it is healthy and fresh, grown in a good soil, grown organically, and in a suitable environment and weather conditions etc. It is a bit like wine making in that there are good and bad years from a particular crop depending on all these conditions.

Second, the extraction method originally used, e.g. distillation. Even with a good quality organically grown plant you can end up with a low quality essential oil if the extraction method was poor. Therefore trained specialists ('Noses' as they are called) are used to assess whether an essential oil meets all the requirements to define its stated qualities. Chemical analysis (by GLC: Gas liquid Chromatography) can be used to check that the oil has not been adulterated by having had chemical additives mixed in. Sadly, a large proportion of essential oils on the market is of a low grade quality and this reduces their therapeutic effect.

CHEMOTYPES (CT)

Chemotypes (CT) is a term used in Aromatherapy to describe the same species of plant but grown in different areas. For example lavender (*Lavandula Angustifolia*) has various different chemotypes, such as high altitude lavender, French Provence lavender and Bulgarian lavender. Although they are all the same species of plant, they have been grown in different environments. The nature of the soil, altitude and the amount of sunshine result in very distinctive variants of essential oil. Chemotypes are often specifically used by experienced aromatherapists with great ensuing benefits because each chemotype has a different therapeutic effect.

CARRIER OILS (Vegetable oils or base oils)

Because pure essential oils can sometimes irritate the skin, they may need to be diluted into carrier oils. A carrier oil also provides lubrication and allows the essential oil to be spread around the body when used in massage. A carrier oil can be almost any pure, high quality, vegetable oil but cold pressed oils are better. Grapeseed, sweet almond, safflower, soya, sunflower and sesame, all make good carriers. Some carrier oils may also be used for their therapeutic effect in their own right: for example peach kernel, avocado and apricot kernel are good for ageing and dry skin, olive oil has many healing properties, and wheatgerm (often added as it is a natural antioxidant to help keep the oils fresh) is good for healing scars on the skin.

FLORAL WATERS

Floral waters or flower waters are a powerful way to use the therapeutic qualities of essential oils without needing the precaution necessary when using the highly concentrated essential oils. Floral waters share all the same therapeutic properties of essential oils and can be applied in very similar ways but they can be used **undiluted** in endless ways - for example:

- As a powerful face wash or cleanser.
- In cooking as flavouring or as a medicinal additive.
- To make delicious medicinal hot or cold drinks.
- With babies in their baths or straight onto their skin thus avoiding any danger of getting the concentrated essential oils in their eyes.
- To moisturise skin and induce powerful therapeutic effects.
- In hot and cold compresses.
- As a mouthwash for sore throats etc.

Floral waters are made in three main ways.

By steam distillation. However, with this method, because they are only a by-product of producing essential oils, not much attention is usually paid to their quality with the consequence that the floral waters often smell burnt and unpleasant. Nevertheless, on occasion, such floral waters can be very good quality.

By alcohol distillation, Here the essential oil is mixed with alcohol and added to water. The alcohol allows the essential oils to completely dissolve into the water. The alcohol is then boiled off. The advantage of this method is that while essential oils do not dissolve in water, they do dissolve in alcohol. However, a disadvantage is that alcohol, as well as the boiling process, can corrupt the oils.

By spring water diffusion. In this, the purest method, essential oil is added to spring water and the mixture left for some weeks, months or even longer so that they impart their properties to the water. The mixture is then filtered to remove the essential oil. This produces a powerful pure floral water with all the properties of essential oil in a safe form.

HOW ESSENTIAL OILS WORK

Essential oils are made up of a complex mixture of different ingredients. Many oils contain hundreds of components often in minute quantities. Each of these components may have a different therapeutic effect. For example Lavender oil contains over 200 different components which may explain why it can be either stimulating, deeply soothing or relaxing, depending on the need of the user.

When an essential oil comes into contact with the body, it passes through the skin (or membranes of the lungs if inhaled) to be absorbed into the blood stream. At this point it soon has a powerful effect on the whole chemistry of the body. These effects are numerous from antiviral to antidepressant. A simple experiment can illustrate this process: if you rub raw garlic onto the sole of your foot it can be smelt on your breath 15 minutes later.

The essential oil Tea-Tree has recently been introduced into the West and is attracting much research into its unique properties. Recent scientific studies have shown that it is effective against all the main varieties of infectious organisms - bacteria, viruses, fungi - as well as being a powerful immune stimulant thereby helping the response and resistance to infection.

The skin can absorb many substances much more efficiently than the lining of the stomach, which is why so many new drugs are being administered through the skin using patches rather than by the more traditional method of swallowing pills. The acidity of the gastric juices in the stomach often ihterfere with drugs taken internally. Indeed, there is a school of thought that you should not put <u>any</u> substance on you skin which is not either natural or edible.

There is not yet an absolute scientific explanation for the therapeutic effects of essential oils in Aromatherapy. Many books and articles have been written on the subject and much research is being carried out today on the pharmacology of essential oils. To know that these oils are indeed therapeutic is far more important than understanding exactly how or why they work.

HOLISTIC AROMATHERAPY

Aromatherapy can be described as truly holistic (working on the whole person), as it simultaneously affects physical, emotional, mental, and spiritual well-being. One of the major advantages of Aromatherapy is its powerful therapeutic action with few, if any, unwanted side effects. Essential oils work in harmony with the body's immune system by assisting the healing process on all levels. It is as if nature had designed these essential oils specifically to work with and heal the body. What an inspiring and comforting idea.

Aromatherapy oils have been used in religious and spiritual ceremonies for many centuries. Frankincense oil has been found to slow the breath and calm the mind making it perfect for a deep prayer and meditation.

For further reading into the subtle and spiritual effects of oils there is a wonderful book by Patricia Davies called 'Subtle Aromatherapy' (see Recommended Further Reading).

HOW TO USE ESSENTIALS OILS AT HOME

One of the great joys of using essential oils, rather than drugs and chemicals, is the knowledge that one can safely treat many conditions without harmful side effects. Although essential oils can be used for their scent or cosmetic qualities, this book is mainly concerned with their medicinal ones.

Please remember that before using a highly concentrated essential oil directly on your skin, you **must** dilute it in a 'carrier' (base/vegetable oil). The most popular carrier oils are sweet almond, grapeseed, and wheatgerm (in small quantities); however any pure vegetable oil will do. To dilute add 20-60 drops of the essential oil to 100 ml of carrier oil (for lesser quantities add 4-15 drops for 25 ml or 3-5 drops for each tablespoon of a carrier oil).

BATHS

From the earliest times baths have been enjoyed. This was so with the Babylonians, ancient Greeks and Romans and, of course, applies to us today. Baths are the easiest and, perhaps, the most pleasurable way of using essential oils. Add 5 to 10 drops of your chosen oils into your bath and stir the water to mix them together. Then soak in the bath for 10 minutes and use this time to relax and take a few deep gentle breaths, light a candle, and enjoy yourself! Such baths deeply nourish the whole self.

If your skin happens to be rather dry, then blend 5-10 drops of the essential oil with 2 teaspoonfuls of base oil and avoid using soaps or body shampoos for the first 5 or 10 minutes to allow time the for the oils to be absorbed into your skin.

Camomile or Lavender are excellent for stress, anxiety, or insomnia.
Rosemary or Pine cure aching limbs and sore muscles.
Ylang Ylang lets you enjoy a euphoric aromatic experience.

If all you want is a **foot or hand bath**, then add 2 to 3 drops of essential oil to a large bowl of hot water. Soak your hands or feet in it for ten to fifteen minutes and enjoy feeling soothed and revived. This is an excellent remedy for tiredness after a long day standing upright or after strenuous exercise. Baths can be combined with almost any other form of health treatment.

HAIR CARE

Hair can be your crowning glory. Add a few drops of essential oil to your final hair rinse or conditioner or just add them directly to any ready made shampoo. This is a very simple way to transform shampoos into deeply nourishing treatments. Your hair and scalp will become full of vitality. Such treatment is very effective for dry scalp conditions and lifeless hair. For conditioning treatment for any type of hair, mix the essential oil in the proportion of 30 - 60 drops to 100 -200 ml of olive oil and/or sweet almond oil. Massage this into the scalp and then wrap the hair in a warm towel for 1 to 2 hours. Rosemary and Camomile condition and encourage healthy hair growth. Bergamot and Tea-Tree are effective in controlling dandruff.

MASSAGE

Massage is a vital part of Aromatherapy because it provides you with the most effective way of applying essential oils to the body. The skin absorbs these oils very readily, and when the whole body is massaged, the essential oils are absorbed into the blood stream in a fairly short time.

Essential oil massages can be deeply relaxing, refreshing, sensuous, muscle toning, and stimulating.

Specific essential oils are chosen to suit the condition and temperament of the user, and then blended with a base oil, such as sweet almond oil or grapeseed oil. Aromatherapists are highly trained in choosing the most appropriate oils.

For general well-being you can massage specific parts of your body, such as your feet or hands. It can also help to rub those parts of the body that are causing discomfort. This will induce a natural healing process.

SKIN OILS AND LOTIONS

Mix a few drops of essential oil into a bland cream or lotion, or add them to a basic face mask, perhaps including oatmeal, honey and pulp from various fruits. A gentle circular movement of the fingers is all that is needed for the oil to be absorbed. This will transform your creams and lotions into powerful healing agents.

STEAM INHALATION

This method is especially suited to sinus, throat and chest infections. Add about 5 drops of an oil such as Peppermint or Thyme to a bowl of boiling-hot water, then cover the head and bowl with a towel and deeply inhale the steam for a minute or so; then, after a pause, repeat the process several times. This allows the essential oils to enter directly into the lungs and respiratory system. They will relieve pain and have a very strong antibacterial and antiviral effect. Steam inhalation is also extremely effective in relieving and healing the symptoms of colds, flu, soar throats and ear infections.

HOT AND COLD COMPRESSES

Compresses are used to relieve pain and reduce inflammation. Even chronic arthritic pains have been relieved in this way as well as injuries, muscle pains, sprains, back pains, and stomach-aches etc.

Hot compresses are made by filling a bowl with very hot water, then adding 4 or 5 drops of essential oil. Soak a piece of plain cotton wool or any other absorbent material large enough to cover the area being treated. Squeeze out the excess water, place over the affected area and secure it by wrapping it in cling film, cloth, or a bandage. Leave the compress on until it has cooled and repeat when necessary. Cold compresses are made in a similar way, using ice-cold water.

VAPORISATION (Room Burner, Oil Burner)

This is a marvellous way to create a harmonious and healing atmosphere in a room. Place a few drops of oil in an essential oil candle burner, a light bulb ring or just add them to a small bowl of water placed on a radiator. Essential oils can change the atmosphere of your home and help calm and soothe places of stress. For example use them in healing and meditation rooms, hospitals and offices.

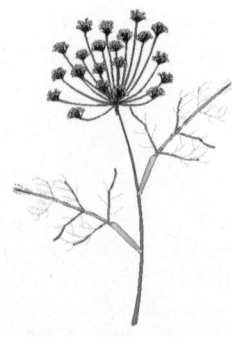

WARNINGS

Never use essential oils directly on your skin.

Keep oils away from the mouth and eyes. If oil should get into the eyes, then wash them with plenty of water or milk.

Store oils in a cool place in dark bottles, close the cap tightly after using.

Keep essential oils out of the reach of children.

Never use more than the suggested or prescribed amounts.

Some essentials oils can irritate the skin and should not be used undiluted in baths. See 'The Essential Oils' section under each oil for details of irritant oils.

Never use essential oils undiluted when bathing babies and young children because they can easily get into their eyes if they rub them with their hands. Always dilute oils in a base (vegetable) oil, such as almond or grapeseed, before adding to the bath. Flower waters are a good alternative to use with babies and children.

Never take essential oils internally. Do not swallow them. If they are accidentally swallowed, drink plenty of milk and consult your doctor.

If you are pregnant, only use Essential Oils in consultation with a qualified Aromatherapist. During the whole of pregnancy avoid Basil, Cinnamon, Cedarwood, Clarysage, Clove, Cypress, Fennel, Hyssop, Jasmine, Juniper, Marjoram, Myrrh, Peppermint and Sage. During the first four months of pregnancy avoid Lavender, Rosemary, Rose and Thyme. Thereafter use these oils only if advised by a professional practitioner.

The following oils may discolour the skin if it is exposed to strong sunlight: Bergamot, Grapefruit, Juniper, Lemon and Mandarin.

If you suffer from epilepsy avoid Fennel, Hyssop, Sage and Wormwood.

If you have high blood pressure avoid Hyssop, Rosemary, Sage and Thyme.

Do not use essential oils during Chemotherapy (seek professional advice).

AN A-Z OF COMMON AILMENTS

ALWAYS CONSULT A MEDICAL DOCTOR BEFORE TREATING ANY SERIOUS CONDITION. THE SUGGESTIONS BELOW WILL ASSIST RATHER THAN REPLACE A MEDICAL TREATMENT.

GENERAL
Aromatherapy oils are often more effective in combination rather than singly. If you prefer, mix together some of the suggested essential oils (See Synergistic Blends in the 'How Essential Oils Are Obtained" section). Oils that are marked with an asterisk (*) make powerful synergistic blends.

The main methods of using essential oils for Aromatherapy purposes are:

- **Baths** : 5-10 drops of essentaial oil added to the bath water and then mixed well.
- **Massage** : 7-25 drops of essential oil in 25 ml (5 tablespoons) of carrier oil (vegetable oil).
- **Inhalations** : 5-10 drops of essential oil in boiling water. Then breathe the steam in deeply while covering the head with a towel.
- **Compresses (hot and cold)** : 5-10 drops of essential oil.
- **Douches** : 1-3 drops of essential oil diluted in a bowl of warm water and bath the affected area.
- **Mouthwash:** Use floral waters or mix about 30 drops of Sage, Thyme, Tea-Tree and Myrrh oils in 100ml of vodka or brandy. Add 2-3 table spoons of this mixture to a glass of water and gargle around mouth. This is an excellent mouth disinfectant and also protects the gums and teeth.

Abscesses and Boils
Bergamot*, Camomile, Lavender*, Tea-Tree*.
Bath, massage, compress, dab with cotton wool.
An abscess or boil often appears when the body is run down due to stress, illness, bad diet etc. They are caused by the body trying to rid itself of impurities or toxins. Apply neat Lavender oil on the infected area. Drink plenty of fluid and eat fresh fruit and vegetables to purify the system. As well as having a strong antibacterial action, these oils help speed up the healing of the infection.

Acne
Bergamot, Camomile, Lavender*, Sandalwood*, Tea-Tree*.
Massage, bath, or apply neat to the skin.
As with boils, it is important to purify the body of toxins through diet and exercise. Drinking plenty of liquid and eating fresh fruit and vegetables is vital. These essential oils are very effective in treating acne due to their powerful antibacterial properties.

A-Z OF COMMON COMPLAINTS

Addictions
Clary Sage*, Rose*, Juniper*, Fennel.
Bath, massage, room burner.
Essential oils can be used to treat the physical and psychological causes of addiction. They can also help overcome the withdrawal symptoms of depression, anger, apathy and physical pain. Be it nicotine or more addictive substances, Clary Sage is particularly effective in overcoming the sense of powerlessness and loss. It's good to experiment to find the oil that suits you. Good luck !

Ageing skin
Neroli*, Lavender*, Jasmine, Geranium, Rose*, Frankincense, Camomile. (Good base oils are avocado, jojoba)
Massage, creams and lotions.
As skin ages, it loses its ability to produce its own oil or sebum and therefore looks dry and more wrinkled. Essential oils stimulate the production of sebum as well as promoting the growth of new cells. Neroli and Lavender are particularly useful in inducing a more vital-looking skin.

Aids (HIV)
Tea-Tree, Lavender, Eucalyptus, Rosemary, Thyme.
Massage, bath, burner, compress.
AIDS itself cannot be treated or cured by Aromatherapy essential oils. Yet with permission from your doctor these oils can be used to help the secondary symptoms and illnesses associated with AIDS. Again, Aromatherapy is not to be used as an alternative to an orthodox treatment but in support or association with it. Most oils are helpful in stimulating the body's natural ability to fight infections. See under individual symptoms.

Allergies
Camomile*, Lavender*, Patchouli, Melissa.
Bath, massage, compress.
Diet and environment play a large role in treating allergies. Essential oils can be used to reduce stress by increasing the body's resistance to whatever is causing the allergic reaction. Melissa and Lavender are very effective in reducing stress and are good for skin allergies. See also under Asthma, Eczema, Hay fever and Stress.

Alopecia (temporary baldness)
Rosemary*, Lavender*, Thyme*.
Massage, compress.
Shock, stress, anxiety, illness and hereditary factors are the main causes of baldness. These oils stimulate the scalp cells.

A-Z of Common Complaints

Anaemia
Camomile*, Lemon, Peppermint, Rosemary*.
Bath, massage, inhalation.

Anger
Rose*, Ylang Ylang, Lavender*.
Bath, massage.
These oils may be stimulating or soothing, depending on the need of the body. Anger is an essential emotion when used with integrity. To suppress anger is as damaging to the body as to lose one's temper all the time.

Anorexia Nervosa
Bergamot*, Lavender*, Camomile, Neroli, Ylang Ylang, Clary Sage*.
Bath, massage.
These oils have a strong uplifting effect on the emotions of the body and stimulate the desire to eat. Always consult a professional practitioner when treating acute conditions.

Anxiety
Lavender*, Frankincense*, Bergamot*, Neroli.
Bath, massage, room burner.
These oils have a soothing and calming effect on the mind and body. Yoga, meditation and deep breathing are very helpful in deepening an understanding of one's fear or anxiety.

Apathy
Lemon*, Cedarwood*, Mandarin*, Jasmine.
Bath, massage.
Stimulates the body and mind. Helps to connect with one's inner purpose.

Aphrodisiac
Sandalwood, Rose*, Jasmine*, Neroli*.
Bath, massage, room burner.
These oils have been traditionally used in folklore as aphrodisiacs. They do have a powerful effect and can help reduce marital tensions, impotence, and frigidity. They certainly make one feel more relaxed and at ease, allowing a deeper and more intimate connection with one's loved one. Use in a room burner or bath to make a lovely atmosphere and aroma, light some candles and create a beautiful space for love.

Appetite (loss of)
Bergamot*, Camomile*, Fennel, Peppermint, Clary Sage.
Bath, compress, massage, room burner.
These oils help stimulate the digestive system and appetite.

A-Z OF COMMON COMPLAINTS

Arthritis
Camomile*, Juniper, Lavender*, Lemon, Marjoram, Rosemary*, Ginger.
Bath, compress, massage, rub the affected area.
To help with arthritis it is essential to look at the person from a holistic point of view. These essential oils are effective in removing toxins from the body (as is a whole-food cleansing diet). They assist in clearing excess uric acid crystals that build up in arthritic joints. Diet and exercise are also important factors in treating this condition. (See Meir Schnieder's book under 'Recommended Further Reading' for more information on effective exercises - page 60).

Asthma
Cedarwood, Clary Sage*, Cypress, Eucalyptus, Frankincense*, Lavender*, Lemon, Marjoram.
Bath, compress, massage, room burner.
Avoid steam inhalations.
The antispasmodic effect of these oils assist in dilating the bronchi (air passages) in the lungs and consequently aid breathing. They also reduce stress and muscle tension. There is usually a complex mixture of causes involved, such as lifestyle, diet and exercise.

Athlete's Foot
Lavender*, Myrrh*, Lemon, Tea-Tree*.
Foot bath, dab with cotton wool.
These oils have a strong antifungal and antiviral action. Apply them on the affected area daily, and the condition usually clears up in one to two weeks.

Babies
Lavender*, Camomile*, Mandarin*.
Essential oils and floral waters are very effective in treating various conditions in little ones. Floral waters can be put straight into baths or onto a baby's skin and are a good alternative to essential oils themselves. When using oils, always dilute them before adding to a bath to avoid any concentrated oil contacting the eyes (1 to 2 drops of essential oil to 10ml of pure vegetable oil, such as grapeseed oil, corn oil or sunflower oil, is sufficient). A drop of Lavender oil on a pillow or night clothes is an effective way of aiding **sleep**. **Colic** is helped by massaging 2 drops of Camomile or Lavender, diluted in 20ml vegetable oil, into the tummy. Camomile is very helpful in **teething:** massage gently around the face to reduce inflammation and pain (use 1 drop 10 ml of oil). For **Fretfulness** or **crying** spells use 2 drops of Geranium and 2 drops of Camomile diluted in vegetable oil, and gently massage the whole body commencing with the feet. This will soothe and calm the baby. For **sickness** and **vomiting** use 1 drop of Peppermint oil to 20ml of vegetable oil and gently rub onto the tummy. For other conditions see under individual headings but always lower the concentration of essential oils.

A-Z OF COMMON COMPLAINTS

Base oil See Carrier oil

Baths (See section '**How to Use Essential Oils at Home**' - page 16)

Blisters
Benzoin*, Lavender*.
Dab with cotton wool.
Allow the blisters to breathe. These oils have an antiseptic effect. They also aid regeneration of the skin.

Blood Pressure See High blood Pressure and Low Blood Pressure

Boils See Abscess

Breathing See Circulation

Bronchitis
Cedarwood, Eucalyptus, Frankincense*, Lavender*, Lemon, Myrrh, Rosemary*, Sandalwood.
Bath, inhalation, massage, rub the chest with massage oil.
Bronchitis often follows a cold, sore throat or flu. It is an infection of the lungs causing the inflammation of the bronchial tubes. Excess mucus production is usually the main factor in aggravating this condition: the lungs being unable to rid themselves of this excess mucus provide a good place for bacteria and viruses to live. These essential oils are effective expectorants, thereby reducing mucus levels. It is also advisable to substitute mucus-forming foods, such as processed foods, white flour, dairy products, and refined starches, with a whole food diet. Steam inhalations are a particularly effective method of introducing the essential oils directly into the lungs, throat and nose.

Bruises
Camomile*, Lavender*.
Bath, compress, dab with cotton wool.
In the later stages of bruises, Rosemary is helpful in stimulating blood circulation around the bruise.

Burns
Eucalyptus*, Lavender*.
Bath, compress.
Lavender is one of the most effective treatments for burns. It can be applied neat directly onto the burnt skin. It will immediately reduce the inflammation and act as an analgesic and antiseptic. *(See under History of Aromatherapy" section about Dr. Gattefosse - page 9.)*

A-Z OF COMMON COMPLAINTS

CANDIDA (albicans)
Tea-Tree*, Myrrh*.
Bath, compress, massage, douches.
These oils have a powerful antifungal agent which will keep in check the candida growth in the digestive system and rest of the body. They are effective in treating vaginal and genital-urinal infections.

CARRIER OILS (Vegetable oils or base oils) See Carrier oils in the '**How Essential Oils Are Obtained**' section - page 13.

CATARRH
Cedarwood, Eucalyptus, Thyme*, Tea-Tree*, Lavender*.
Bath, steam inhalation, face-massage.
These oils are effective in clearing the nasal and respiratory passages as well as being strong antibacterial and antiviral agents. It is important to look at diet when the body is producing too much catarrh or mucus. Avoiding dairy products and wheat can be helpful. Try consulting a nutritionist.

CELLULITE
Fennel, Geranium*, Rosemary*.
Bath, massage, rub with massage oil.
Essential oils are very helpful in treating cellulite which can often be related to hormonal imbalance and diet. The need to detoxify the body and harmonise the hormonal system is important. Geranium contains a plant hormone which helps balance the body's endocrine or hormonal system.

CHICKEN POX
Tea-Tree*, Bergamot*, Camomile*.
Bath, gentle massage, room burner.
These antiviral oils are effective in helping to heal this condition. Camomile helps reduce itching and aids sleeping.

CHILBLAINS also see under CIRCULATION
Cypress*, Lavender*, Lemon, Sandalwood.
Bath, compress.
Chilblains are a sign of poor circulation: these oils will help stimulate the circulation. Shallow breathing slows down the whole circulatory system. Yoga and stretching help stimulate the circulation as does more aware breathing.

CHILDBIRTH
Jasmine*, Lavender*, Neroli*, Rose*.
Bath, compress, massage.
To encourage and strengthen contractions use Jasmine and Lavender which are also analgesic (pain relieving). These have been used safely with great success by many women to help the uterus muscles relax and to soothe pain during contractions. Massage the oils over the whole abdomen and back. Neroli helps calm and relax emotions and breathing; it is also uplifting.

A-Z of Common Complaints

CHILDREN also see under BABIES.
Lavender*, Rose*, Benzoin, Mandarin.
Bath, compress, inhalation, massage.
Essential oils are very useful with children, who respond quickly to treatments. However, a few cautions need to be observed; always dilute oils: use half or quarter concentrations (1 drop of essential oil in 2 table spoons of vegetable oil); never use oils internally.

CHILLINESS also see under CIRCULATION
Cypress, Lavender*, Frankincense*, Rosemary*.
Bath, compress, inhalation, massage.
These oils help stimulate the whole circulation thereby warming the body. If prone to getting cold, it is important to increase the efficiency of the circulation.

CIRCULATION
Juniper, Rosemary*, Marjoram*. (Garlic, tablets or fresh).
Bath, compress, inhalation, massage.
All these oils help stimulate circulation, which is vital for good health. When circulation is poor, the blood cannot flow efficiently, with the result that the body does not receive enough oxygen or nutrients. This in turn causes tiredness and a weak immune system. It is important to increase the efficiency of your circulation by breathing more deeply, and with greater awareness. It is very common for people not to breathe deeply enough thereby depriving the body of oxygen and life-force. Yoga, stretching, massage, and regular exercise all help to reduce muscle tension which inhibits proper breathing.

COLDS
Cypress, Eucalyptus*, Tea-Tree*, Lavender*, Thyme*.
Bath, steam inhalation.
These oils contain powerful antiviral agents. A cold is caused by a virus which affects the upper respiratory area of the nose and throat. Inhalations are very helpful as they carry the essential oil directly into the throat, nose and lungs to soothe and fight the infection. Lavender aids sleep and is an analgesic. Vitamin C and garlic also help. Avoid mucus-forming foods (dairy-products, bread etc.).

COLD SORES (herpes simplex 1)
Bergamot, Eucalyptus*, Lavender*, Tea-Tree*.
Dab with cotton wool at the outset of the infection to prevent blisters from forming. Lavender can be applied undiluted or the oils can be mixed with alcohol (6 drops to 5 ml to alcohol) and dabbed onto the sores regularly.

COLIC see BABIES

COMPRESSES (HOT AND COLD) See section 'How To Use Essential Oils at home' - page 18.

A-Z OF COMMON COMPLAINTS

Confidence (lack of)
Ylang Ylang*, Bergamot*.
Bath, massage, room burner.
These oils uplift the spirit and emotions and also have a strong antidepressant effect.

Conjunctivitis
Flower/floral waters (Never put essential oils directly on the eyes).
Compress over infected eye at night.
Using herbs in the compress is helpful. A convenient method is to place a lukewarm moist camomile tea bag over the eye to soothe and for an antiviral action. Bathe the eye with floral waters.

Constipation
Marjoram*, Fennel, Rosemary*, Mandarin.
Bath, massage, rub the abdomen with massage oil.
Massage the oils around the abdomen to stimulate the digestive tract. Adopt a diet of unrefined carbohydrates, fruit and raw vegetable juices. Drink plenty of liquids. Reduce stress levels with meditation, yoga, and exercise.

Convalescence
Bath, compress, inhalation, massage.
Rosemary*, Bergamot*, Clary Sage*.
These oils stimulate the immune system and help the body regain its strength. It is important to follow a whole food diet, take regular exercise within one's own ability, and to rest. This applies to both minor and major conditions, from flu to a major surgery.

Coughs
Eucalyptus, Thyme*, Lavender*, Benzoin*, Sandalwood, Tea-Tree*.
Massage, steam inhalations. Floral waters are good to gargle with and soothe the throat.
Benzoin is particularly soothing for the throat. Thyme and Tea-Tree are both very powerful antiviral/bacterial agents. Inhalations carry the essential oil in the steam directly into the throat, nose and lungs. Lavender aids sleep as it is an analgesic, and reduces inflammation. Vitamin C, garlic and avoiding mucus-forming foods are also helpful.

Courage (lack of)
Frankincense, Sandalwood, Rose*, Ylang Ylang*.
Bath, inhalation, massage.
These oils have an uplifting effect on the emotions and spirit. Ylang Ylang is a stimulant, an antidepressant and has euphoric effects. Frankincense calms and soothes.

A-Z OF COMMON COMPLAINTS

Cramp
Juniper, Lavender*, Rosemary*.
Bath, massage, rub with massage oil.
These help stimulate the circulatory system. Rosemary is particularly helpful.

Cuts
Lavender*, Tea-Tree*.
Compress, dab drops on cotton wool and apply directly to the cut.
As antiseptic lotions, essential oils are very good in helping heal cuts and are good alternatives to TCP or surgical spirit in the medicine cupboard. (They have the ability to kill all bacteria without damaging the body tissue, unlike normal antiseptics which kill both the body tissue and bacteria. This is partly why they sting so much!).

Cystitis
Eucalyptus, Bergamot*, Juniper, Lavender*, Sandalwood.
Hot compress, massage the abdomen with massage oil.
Cystitis is an inflammation of the bladder usually caused by bacteria. It is more common in women as the female urethra is much shorter than in men, making it easier for bacteria to reach the bladder. Bergamot (using very low dilutions of around 1% or 1-2 drops per 100 ml of warm water) can be used with a douche or external wash. Also drink plenty of liquid, especially camomile tea.

Dandruff
Cypress*, Cedarwood, Rosemary*, Mandarin.
Scalp massage, hair tonic.
These oils stimulate the blood flow in the scalp and help keep the skin moist and flexible. Add these oils to your conditioner or shampoo.

Deodorant
Bergamot, Lavender, Neroli.
Mix in flower water or use a room or candle burner.
These oils are all effective body deodorants.

Depression
For calming use **Camomile*, Clary Sage, Lavender*, Ylang Ylang, Sandalwood.**
For restlessness use **Bergamot*, Jasmine, Geranium*.**
Bath, inhalation, massage.
These oils all have the ability to uplift the spirits and help us connect with the lighter, happier parts of ourselves.

Dermatitis
Cypress*, Geranium*, Juniper, Lavender*, Patchouli.
Bath, compress, apply oil to an affected area.

A-Z OF COMMON COMPLAINTS

Detoxifying
Juniper*, Lavender*, Geranium, Rosemary*.
Bath, massage.
These oils can help eliminate toxins by their diuretic effect; they also stimulate the circulation. This process can be assisted by adopting a cleansing diet.

Diarrhoea
Camomile*, Cypress, Eucalyptus, Lavender*, Neroli.
Massage, compress, floral water to take internally.
Eucalyptus is the most effective if a viral or bacterial cause is suspected. Camomile is good when there is an allergic reaction. If stress or anxiety is the cause, then Lavender, Camomile and Neroli are helpful. It is important to drink plenty of water and herbal teas, such as camomile, and to eat lightly.

Douche see beginning of this section.

Earache (Otitis)
Camomile, Lavender.
Cotton wool in the ear with a drop of massage oil. Hot compress around the ear. Steam inhalation.
Make sure the eardrum is not perforated before doing this: pour a teaspoon of warm almond oil mixed with 3 drops of above oils into the ear, insert a cotton wool plug, and then leave for half an hour. Always consult your doctor because ear infections need to be treated with a great caution, due to the potential risk of spreading the infection. If earaches reoccur, it is important to prevent congestion from too much mucus when the body overproduces catarrh. Avoid dairy products and wheat. Try consulting a nutritionist.

Eczema
Camomile*, Frankincense*, Bergamot, Melissa (low dilution), Lavender*.
Bath, apply massage oil to affected areas.
Some eczemas are stress-related, others are caused by allergic reaction. Try mixing Camomile and Melissa in a pure unscented moisturising or aqueous cream. Avoid processed or refined food and watch out for allergic reactions to dust and animals.

Exhaustion
Clary Sage*, Lavender*, Frankincense, Thyme*.
Bath, massage, inhalations.
These oils are soothing and relaxing, whereas Eucalyptus and Thyme are stimulating.

A-Z OF COMMON COMPLAINTS

Fainting
Peppermint*, Neroli, Basil, Lavender*, Rosemary*.
Bath, massage, room burner. Or hold the bottle, or drops, on a tissue under the nose.
Dr. Bach's Rescue remedy is also very good. If fainting regularly reoccurs then consult your doctor to check on blood pressure etc.

Fatigue
Thyme*, Rosemary*, Lavender*, Geranium*.
Bath massage, room burner.
These oils are all stimulants. Rosemary is also a mind as well as a body stimulant. Lavender and Geranium are more calming and balancing.

Fear
Frankincense*, Sandalwood, Rose*, Ylang Ylang.
Bath, compress, massage, room burner.
These oils are deeply soothing and calming in times of stress and fear.

Fever
Basil, Camomile*, Cypress, Lavender*, Rosemary, Peppermint, Bergamot, Eucalyptus.
Gently massage the back or sponge the forehead with water mixed with oils.
These oils induce and encourage sweating thereby speeding up the healing process. Many viruses cannot survive when the body temperature is above normal. However, if the temperature should rise above 102-103° F it is advisable to try and reduce the temperature. Bergamot, Eucalyptus, Peppermint, and Lavender all have a cooling effect, and help to reduce the fever. These oils are effective when the fever is dangerously high and especially so with babies and children. Always consult a doctor when the fever is high or prolonged.

Flatulence
Camomile*, Fennel*, Peppermint*, Rosemary, Mandarin.
Massage on the abdomen.
These oils help calm the digestive system and are antispasmodic. When flatulence is a constant problem, it is important to look carefully at one's diet. Common causes are insufficient chewing or eating too quickly.

Fleas see Lice

Floral waters (or flower waters)
See under Floral waters in the 'How Essential Oils Are Obtained' section.

A-Z OF COMMON COMPLAINTS

Flu (Influenza)
Eucalyptus*, Thyme*, Frankincense, Ginger, Lavender*, Peppermint, Tea-Tree*.
Bath, compress, massage, inhalation.
Having a hot bath using Tea-Tree oil or steam inhalation with some of the above oils will often completely halt the spread of flu viruses or else shorten the length of the infection. Lavender has strong analgesic properties and aids sleep. Tea -Tree and Eucalyptus are very powerful antiviral agents.

Fluid retention
Eucalyptus, Geranium*, Lavender*, Lemon grass, Rosemary, Thyme, Cypress*.
Bath, massage.
Cypress oil is particularly effective when there is too much fluid in the body causing weight gain or swelling joints. Exercises like yoga or stretches are also helpful.

Frigidity
Clary Sage, Neroli*, Jasmine*, Patchouli, Rose*, Sandalwood*, Ylang Ylang.
Bath, massage, room burner.
Luxurious oils, such as Rose and Jasmine, are particularly related to female sexuality. They give a sense of self-worth and beauty. These essential oils help deepl relaxation and letting go of tension, therefore helping with frigidity and fear. Although these oils are very expensive, they are potent and so only small amounts are needed.

Gall stones
Lavender*, Rosemary*.
Massage, bath.
Gall stones are often a solidified cholesterol, therefore animal fats should be reduced in one's diet.

Gingivitis (Gum inflammation)
Sage, Thyme, Tea-Tree, Myrrh.
Mouth wash. Floral waters are effective as a mouth wash.

Gout (See Arthritis)
Juniper*, Lemon, Rosemary*.
Foot bath, compress, massage.

Grief
Melissa*, Frankincense*, Marjoram, Rose*, Mandarin.
Bath, massage, room burner.
Rose oil is particularly warming and soothing. Melissa is very good for deep grief. It is important to get support and help from a caring person. This is where massage combined with Aromatherapy is so helpful.

A-Z OF COMMON COMPLAINTS

GUMS see GINGIVITIS

HAEMORRHOIDS (Piles)
Cypress*, Frankincense*.
Bath, general massage.
Haemorrhoids are varicose veins in the rectum. These oils will assist in increasing blood circulation. Regular exercise is also important as are yoga, stretches and learning to breath more deeply. (See Circulation).

HAIR LOSS see ALOPECIA
Lavender, Rosemary, Ylang Ylang.
Scalp oil. Add 5-10 drops of essential oil to a carrier oil and rub into the hair daily. Oils help to stimulate the scalp.

HAIR CARE see DANDRUFF and in the 'How to Use Essential Oils At Home' section - see page 16.

HANGOVER
Juniper*, Rose, Rosemary*.
Bath, inhalation, massage.
Juniper is particularly effective in cleansing the body of toxins. Drink plenty of water as alcohol dehydrates the body.

HAY FEVER
Juniper, Camomile*, Melissa*, Lavender*.
Inhale from drops on handkerchief, inhalations, massage.
These oils are helpful in two main ways: firstly, they help clear the symptoms of a runny nose, watery eyes, itching and sneezing; and secondly, if used regularly, they have the ability to increase resistance to allergens.

HEADACHE AND MIGRAINE
Clary Sage*, Camomile, Lavender*, Marjoram*, Peppermint, Rose, Rosemary.
Bath, compress, massage or apply oil to the head, neck and shoulder. Room burner.
Lavender is a strong analgesic (gives pain-relief). Rosemary helps increase the blood flow around the head. If headaches are regular, then it is important to look at other factors such as lifestyle, stress levels, diet and exercise. Caffeine and chocolate are two common causes of headaches.

HERPES see COLD SORES

HIGH BLOOD PRESSURE (Hypertension)
Lavender*, Marjoram, Ylang Ylang*.
Massage, inhalations, bath.
These oils have a strong ability to lower the blood pressure by helping the

A-Z OF COMMON COMPLAINTS

body relax and by regulating the sympathetic nervous system. Regular massage with essential oils can reduce blood pressure dramatically. Diet, exercise, yoga and meditation reduce stress and other causes of high blood pressure. It is important to talk to a trained professional for advice to avoid the risks of cardiac conditions, such as strokes and coronary thrombosis.

Hoarseness and loss of voice
Cypress, Lavender*, Sandalwood*.
Bath, compress, massage, rub on the throat and chest.

Homeopathy
Oils to avoid while taking homeopathic medicine are the stronger ones, such as Peppermint, Eucalyptus, Thyme, Rosemary and Sage. However, most oils may be used (always consult your homeopath first as there are many different opinions).

Hysteria
Camomile, Clary Sage*, Lavender*, Bergamot*.
Bath, room burner.
These oils are deeply calming.

Immune System
Camomile, Lavender*, Eucalyptus, Tea-Tree*, Rosemary, Geranium*.
Bath, compress, inhalation, massage.
Besides their antiviral and antibacterial properties, these essential oils actually stimulate the body's immune response to illness. Lavender, Eucalyptus, Bergamot and Tea-Tree particularly combine these two elements. Geranium and Rosemary also assist the adrenal and lymphatic systems to fight against infections. Tea-Tree is probably the single most important oil in this respect. It also has antifungal properties. It is the strongest immune system stimulant I know of. Using essential oils regularly in baths, massage etc. is an effective way of preventing everyday illnesses from occurring. It is essential to look simultaneously at one's lifestyle, diet and exercise patterns.

Indecision
Patchouli, Rosemary*, Thyme*.
Bath massage, room burner.
These oils stimulate the mind thereby allowing one to think more clearly.

Indigestion
Bergamot, Camomile*, Fennel*, Juniper, Lavender*, Lemon, Peppermint, Rosemary, Mandarin.
Bath, massage, compress.
Gently massage the stomach or use a hot compress. Drinking herbal teas (e.g. camomile, fennel, peppermint) also helps soothe the stomach and neutralise acids.

INFLAMMATION
Camomile*, Lavender*, Eucalyptus, Myrrh.
Bath, massage, warm compress.
Camomile is the most effective anti-inflammatory oil that helps both internal and external inflammations, ranging from stomach upsets and infected cuts to arthritis.

INHALATIONS see STEAM INHALATIONS

INSOMNIA
Camomile*, Lavender*, Rose, Sandalwood, Ylang Ylang, Neroli.
Bath, massage, room burner. Few drops on a tissue, near pillow.
Lavender, Camomile and Neroli are particularly effective in calming the mind from the emotions rising from stress and worry. All the oils listed have strong sedative qualities. If insomnia is frequent, it is helpful to learn to use relaxation techniques, meditation, and to do stretches or yoga before going to bed. Massage is also very helpful for reducing stress.

IRRITABILITY
Camomile*, Cypress, Lavender*, Ylang Ylang.
Bath, massage, inhalation.
These oils balance the body, mind and emotions. They encourage expression where suppressed emotions are involved and calm where emotions are uncontrollable. The great gift of natural essential oils is the ability to work in harmony with the body and mind.

JEALOUSY
Rose*, Benzoin, Camomile*.
Bath, massage, inhalation.
These oils have natural sedative and calming affects. They help soothe the emotions.

KIDNEYS
Camomile, Cedarwood*, Juniper*.
Bath, massage.
These oils act as a tonic to the kidneys, helping stimulate and heal their function. However, always consult a medical professional when dealing with such important organs as the kidneys.

LARYNGITIS
Lavender*, Thyme*, Eucalyptus, Benzoin*, Sandalwood.
Bath, compress, steam inhalation, rub oil on the throat and chest.
Benzoin is particularly soothing for the throat.

A-Z OF COMMON COMPLAINTS

Lice
Bergamot, Eucalyptus, Geranium and Lavender all mixed together.
An effective way of getting rid of lice and fleas in children and adults is to add oils to shampoo (around 5-10% or 30-40 drops in 100 ml) or to vegetable oil and massage in the hair, and leave for half an hour and then rinse. Repeat after 48 hours. Or rub the scalp with a mixture of 5 ml of an essential oil to 100 ml of vodka. Remember to wash the garments (clothes, coats, scarves, bedding etc.) where eggs might later hatch.

Liver
Rosemary*, Camomile*, Peppermint.
Massage, bath, inhalations.
Rosemary is a particularly effective stimulant and tonic to the liver. It encourages bile production, and helps jaundice. The liver is the largest organ of the body and has many different functions. It detoxifies the body of pollutants (alcohol, chemicals from food, air pollution etc.) and manufactures bile and vitamin A.

Low blood pressure (Hypotension)
Rosemary*, Black pepper*, Clary Sage*.
Strong massage, hot bath, inhalation.
These oils are effective stimulants and will aid the circulatory system. Low blood pressure is far less common than high blood pressure but can cause dizziness, fainting, coldness etc. It is important to improve the circulatory system. (See Circulation).

Massage
See 'How to Use Essential Oils At Home' section - page 17.

ME
(Myalgic Encephalomyelitis or Chronic Fatigue Syndrome) See under Case Histories section - page 55.

Measles
Eucalyptus*, Tea-Tree*.
Room burner going all the time, bath.
These two oils used together are powerful antiviral agents and immune system stimulants. It is good to gently sponge the forehead with water with essential oils added. Always consult your doctor.

Meditation
see end of Case Histories section - page 59.

Memory
Basil*, Juniper*, Rosemary*.
Bath, inhalation, massage.
These oils all stimulate the central nervous system and the brain. For instance, they help concentration in exams.

35

A-Z OF COMMON COMPLAINTS

Menopause
Camomile, Rose*, Geranium*, Jasmine, Lavender*, Sandalwood.
Bath, inhalation, massage.
Geranium is helpful as it contains a natural plant hormone that helps regulate the hormonal system. Rose balances and tones the uterus and harmonises the menstrual cycle. Camomile is a calming, antidepressant oil. All these oils used together have a strong impact on a difficult menopause. Evening primrose oil and multi-vitamins, especially vitamin B and calcium, are also helpful.

Menstruation.
Cypress*, Geranium*. (For heavy periods)
Clary Sage*, Juniper, Lavender*. (For irregular or painful periods)
Rosemary bath, compress, rub the abdomen with massage oil.
Lavender is helpful for pain-relief and is a good muscle relaxant. Geranium contains a natural plant hormone which helps regulate the hormonal system.

Migraine see Headache

Mood swings
Bergamot, Camomile*, Geranium*, Lavender*.
Bath, massage, room burner.
Geranium is particularly good at balancing moods. Bergamot is an uplifting antidepressant oil.

Mouth wash
Floral waters are very effective (see beginning of the A-Z section - page 20).

Multiple Sclerosis (MS)
See under Case Histories - page 54.

Muscles (aching)
Lavender*, Camomile*, Rosemary*, Marjoram.
All these oils have strong muscle-relaxant properties and Lavender in particular is a strong analgesic.

Nausea (Vomiting) also see Travel sickness
Camomile, Fennel, Lavender*, Peppermint*.
Bath, inhalation, massage, compress on the stomach with warm water.

Nervous tension also see Anxiety, Depression, Stress
Lavender*, Marjoram, Rose*, Sandalwood, Mandarin, Ylang Ylang.
Bath, massage, room burner.

A-Z OF COMMON COMPLAINTS

Neuralgia
Camomile*, Geranium*, Lavender*, Clary Sage, Rosemary.
Bath, compress, rub the affected area with oil.
The intense pain associated with this condition is helped by the analgesic properties of Lavender and Camomile as well as by their anti-inflammatory properties. Cool compresses help soothe the inflamed nerves.

Nosebleeds
Lemon.
Place 1-3 drops of Lemon oil on a cool wet cotton wool and insert into the nose.
Lemon is haemostatic (helps the blood to clot).

Obsessions
Clary Sage*, Frankincense*.
Bath, inhalation, massage.
These oils help calm and sedate emotions.

Pets
Essential oils are very effective in treating animals, e.g. to control fleas and lice, tics etc. Use Eucalyptus., Lavender, Bergamot- these may also be used as an antiseptic for wounds and cuts.

PMT (premenstrual tension) also see Menstruation
Camomile*, Cypress, Geranium*, Rosemary, Lavender, Rose*.
Bath, compress, massage.
These oils reduce stress and anxiety. Geranium helps regulate the hormonal change of the body. Lavender is a natural analgesic.

Pneumonia
Eucalyptus*, Lavender*, Tea-Tree*.
Massage, inhalations, room burner.
Always consult a medical professional when treating this condition. Inhalations are helpful as they carry the essential oil directly into the throat, nose and lungs to soothe and help fight the infection. Lavender aids sleep as it is an analgesic and reduces inflammation. Tea-Tree is a powerful immune system stimulant, helpful in this potentially dangerous condition. Take vitamin C and garlic while avoiding mucus-forming foods (dairy products, bread etc.). Follow a wholefood diet. It is important to allow the body plenty of rest and time to convalesce.

Pregnancy see Childbirth and Warnings section.
AVOID Basil, Cedarwood, Clary Sage, Cypress, Fennel, Jasmine, Juniper, Marjoram, Myrrh, Peppermint, Rose, Rosemary and Thyme.
USE Mandarin, Geranium*, Ylang Ylang, and Lavender*.
All oils should be used in minimum concentrations for safety. Good remedies for morning sickness are herbal teas or Lavender in very small dilution (1 drop to 50 ml) massaged gently around the stomach.

37

A-Z OF COMMON COMPLAINTS

Psoriasis
Bergamot, Geranium*, Juniper*, Lavender*, Tea-Tree.
Bath, compress.
Reducing stress and maintaining a good diet have helped many people with this condition. These oils used are good for dealing with stress and they also stimulate a natural resistance to this difficult condition.

Refreshing
Rosemary, Bergamot*, Lemon*, Lavender*.
Bath, massage.
These uplifting and invigorating oils help one become more alert, energised and clear-headed.

Rejuvenatiion
Frankincense*, Lavender*, Neroli*.
Bath, compress, massage.
Lavender and Neroli are strong cytophilactic oils (they stimulate the growth of new cells in the body and skin). This encourages the body to maintain faster cellular regeneration to compensate for its natural decline with age. Other factors, such as diet, exercise, lifestyle and stress, also play an important role.

Relaxation
Lavender*, Bergamot*, Camomile*.
Bath, massage, room burner.
These oils have a deeply sedative and calming effect on the body and mind. Yoga, meditation and relaxation tapes can also help enormously.

Rheumatism
Camomile*, Eucalyptus, Lavender*, Lemon, Marjoram, Rosemary*.
Bath, compress, massage the affected area with oil.
Lavender and Camomile are strong analgesics while Camomile also has an anti-inflammatory effect. Warm compresses are helpful. Adopting fresh wholefood diet and doing stretching exercises assist in the release of toxins and uric acid.

Room burner
see 'Vaporisation, in the 'How To Use Essential oils At Home' section - page 18.

Scabies
Lavender*, Peppermint*, Rosemary*.
A combination of these oils (5% dilution, 50 drops to 100 ml) added to a normal cream or moisturiser and applied a few times a day is effective in removing these itching beasties. Wash all clothes and bedding.

A-Z OF COMMON COMPLAINTS

Sciatica
Lavender*, Camomile*.
Compresses, massage.
These oils on compresses will reduce the inflammation of the sciatic nerve. Massage is also good when the pain is less acute. Lavender is a strong analgesic.

Sedative
Camomile*, Clary Sage, Lavender*, Bergamot.
Bath, room burner.
These oils are deeply calming.

Shock
Neroli, Melissa, Lavender*, Peppermint*, Rose*, Ylang Ylang.
Bath, massage, room burner.
These oils have a calming effect and soothe the central nervous system. One can apply Lavender neat to the temples or wrists. Rescue remedy from Dr. Bach's is also very useful.

Sinusitis
Tea-Tree*, Thyme, Eucalyptus*, Lavender*.
Bath, inhalation, compress, steam inhalation.
Eucalyptus and Lavender are good decongestants and help with pain relief. Tea-Tree is a strong antiseptic and should be used if sinusitis is accompanied by a cold or any other infection.

Skin problems See Ageing skin, Acne and the 'How To Use Essential Oils At Home' section.
Blotchy - Geranium.   *Chapped* - Benzoin.   *Cracked* - Frankincense.
Dry - Geranium, Sandalwood.   *Inflamed* - Camomile, Clary Sage, Sandalwood, Tea-Tree.
Itchy - Lavender.   *Oily* - Cedarwood, Cypress.
Bath, compress, massage.
Calendular cream is also good. Add essential oils to a normal moisturising cream to make your own remedies. Use about 10 drops of oil in a 100 ml bottle and mix well.

Sore throat see Tonsillitis and Throat infections

Spasm
Camomile*, Clary Sage*, Lavender*.
Massage, bath, compress.
All these oils are strongly antispasmodic.

39

A-Z OF COMMON COMPLAINTS

Sprains
Lavender*, Camomile*.
Compresses.
These oils are strong analgesics.

Steam Inhalations
See the '**How To Use Essential Oils At Home**' section.

Sterility
Geranium*, Rose*, Jasmine*, Neroli*, Bergamot.
Geranium and Rose help balance hormonal functions and have a normalising effect on the female reproductive system. Rose has been known to increase sperm count and therefore can be used by both partners. To help reduce the stress of not being able to conceive, Bergamot, Clary Sage, Jasmine, Neroli and Rose are all used.

Stiffness
Eucalyptus, Lavender*, Marjoram*, Rosemary*.
Bath, massage, compress.
These oils all help muscles relax, while Lavender and Rosemary are also pain relievers.

Stomachache
Fennel, Lavender*, Marjoram, Peppermint, Camomile*.
Bath, massage / rub with massage oil.
Camomile is a strong antispasmodic oil and relaxes the muscles of the digestive system. Muscle cramp is often the cause of stomach pain. Lavender also helps relieve pain.

Stress
Bergamot, Camomile*, Clary Sage*, Jasmine, Lavender*, Marjoram, Neroli, Rose.
Massage, baths, inhalations.
All these oils are deeply relaxing and help relieve tension. Aromatherapy massage is particularly nourishing during times of stress. Yyoga and meditation are also helpful. Long hot baths with lovely oils in them are a great treat. See Meditation at the end of the 'Case History' section.

Sunburn
Camomile*, Lavender*.
Bath, cold compress.
Both these oils have a very soothing and healing effect on the skin. Camomile is soothing and cooling for minor burns and Lavender is good for stronger sunburn. (Also see under Burns.) Add oils to a moisturising cream or carrier oil.

Synergy or Synergistic blends
see the '**How Essential Oils Are Obtained**' section -page 11.

40

A-Z OF COMMON COMPLAINTS

Teething pain
Camomile*, Clove, Peppermint*.
Compress, mouthwash.
Camomile is very helpful when babies are teething. Gently massage babies around the face to reduce the inflammation and pain. (Use 1 drop to 10 ml of oil.)

Thrush see Candida
Tea-Tree*, Myrrh*.
Bath, douche.
Both Myrrh and Tea-Tree are strong antifungal agents and help control this infection.

Tiredness see Fatigue

Tonsillitis and Throat infections
Clary Sage, Eucalyptus, Geranium, Tea-Tree*, Lavender*, Benzoin*, Thyme*.
Bath, compress, rub massage oil on the throat and upper chest, inhalations.
Benzoin is particularly soothing for the throat; Thyme and Tea-Tree are both very powerful antibacterial agents. Inhalations are most helpful as they carry the essential oil in the steam directly into the throat, nose and lungs helping to soothe, and fight the infection. Lavender aids sleep and reduces inflammation. Vitamin C, garlic and avoiding mucus-forming foods (dairy products, bread) also help.

Toothache
Camomile*, Clove, Peppermint, Lavender*.
Compress, mouthwash.
Lavender and Camomile are good pain relievers and help reduce inflammation and infection due to their antiseptic and anti-inflammatory properties.

Travel sickness
Lavender*, Peppermint*.
Sniff a few drops on a tissue or tummy-massage with Camomile and Lavender.
Good for children on long journeys.

Ulcers (mouth)
Myrrh.
Mouth wash.
This oil is particularly effective for mouth ulcers as it works well in damp areas of the body.

Urinary infections see Cystitis
Bergamot*, Cypress, Eucalyptus, Juniper*, Lavender*, Thyme.
Bath, massage/rub onto the abdomen with a massage oil.

A-Z OF COMMON COMPLAINTS

Varicose veins
Cypress*, Lemon, Lavender*.
Bath, compress.
It is very important to improve the circulation of the body, see Circulation.

Vegetable oils see Carrier oils.

Verrucas
Lemon*, Tea-Tree*.
Dab directly with oil.
Verrucas are caused by a virus. Both these oils have a strong antiviral effect. Another treatment is to use a mixture of cider vinegar and <u>Lemon</u> (1 drop of <u>Lemon</u> to 5 drops of cider vinegar), place this on the wart or verruca then cover it with a plaster during the day and leave it open at night.

Viral infections see Coughs, Colds, Sore throat
Tea-Tree*, Bergamot*, Eucalyptus*.
Massage, bath, inhalations, room burner.

Vomiting see Nausea

Warnings see page 19

Warts see Verrucas
Lemon*, Tea-Tree*.
Dab with neat essential oil.

Whooping Cough
Tea-Tree*, Rosemary*, Lavender*, Thyme.
Massage, inhalations, bath.
Steam inhalations are particularly helpful with <u>Tea-Tree</u> and <u>Lavender</u>; they help soothe the throat and ease coughing fits.

Wounds & Sores see Cuts
Lavender, Patchouli, Lemon.
Bath, compress.

Wrinkles see Skin problems & Ageing skin
Clary Sage, Frankincense*, Rose*, Rosemary.
Bath, massage, skin lotions.

* <u>Means Synergistic Blend</u> (see Synergistic Blends in the 'How Essential Oils Are Obtained' Section).

THE ESSENTIAL OILS

The following symbols are used in describing the individual essential oils:

THE OIL *(Latin Name)*
- ◖ The smell and the part of the plant it comes from.
- ☞ The geographic origins. (The first countries listed are the plant's native origin country.)
- ✪ The oil's physical healing qualities.
- ✶ The oil's effect on mind, emotion and spirit.
- ★ Cautions needed when using this oil.
- ⓒ Notes and explanations.

ANGELICA *(Angelica archangelica)*
- ◖ Fresh, spicy, earthy fragrance. Obtained from roots or seed.
- ☞ Europe, Siberia, cultivated mainly in Belgium, Hungary and Germany.
- ✪ Stress, tension, cleanses the body of toxins, good for coughs.
- ✶ Tradionally used to help connect with angels and one's dreams.
- ★ Root oil is phototoxic (seed oil is not). Not to be used during pregnancy or by diabetics.

BASIL *(Ocimum basilicum)*
- ◖ Sweet, herbaceous, camphor odour. Obtained from leaves and flowers.
- ☞ Tropical Asia and Africa. Now cultivated worldwide, especially France, Italy, Egypt, Bulgaria, Hungary, USA.
- ✪ Respiratory infections, tired muscles, soothes the digestive system, clears the mind.
- ★ Mild skin irritant. Avoid during pregnancy.

BAY LAUREL *(laurus nobilis)*
- ◖ Strong, spicy, medicinal odour. Obtained from dried leaves and twigs.
- ☞ Mediterranean, oil obtained largely from eastern Europe.
- ✪ Viral infections, immune system, colds, good for the digestive system, wind.
- ★ Occasional skin sensitivity. Do not use during pregnancy.

BENZOIN *(Styrax benzoin)*
- ◖ Rich, viscous liquid with a sweet vanilla odour. Obtained from resin.
- ☞ Tropical Asia. Main production from Asia.
- ✪ Sore throats, colds, flu, infectious conditions.
- ✶ Helps balance emotions (e.g. anger) and the base or root chakra.

The Essential Oils

Bergamot *(Citrus bergamia)*
- ☻ Refreshing, flowery, citrus flavour. Obtained from rind of fruit.
- ▣ Tropical Asia. Oil obtained from south Italy and the Ivory Coast.
- ☺ Urinary conditions, e.g. cystitis. Good for skin care.
- ☯ Heals the heart, love & grief, depression and anxiety. A strong antidepressant.
- ☹ Do not use before exposing the skin to sunlight or a sun bed. Can discolour the skin when exposed to a very bright light as it reacts with pigments in the skin.

Cajeput *(Melaleuca cajeputi)*
- ☻ Camphor, penetrating odour. Obtained from twigs and leaves.
- ▣ Asia and Australia.
- ☺ Colds, respiratory conditions, revitalising and stimulating.

Camomile roman *(Chamaemelum nobile)*
- ☻ Lovely strong musty smell. Obtained from flowers.
- ▣ Europe. Oil obtained from England, the rest of Europe, USA.
- ☺ Sore throats, sleeping difficulties, insomnia, digestive problems, any inflammation.
- ☯ Soothes anger and calms the mind in stress.
- ☹ Occasional skin irritant.
- 📖 *There are three types of camomile used in Aromatherapy. Roman camomile listed above. German camomile blue (Matriccaria recutica) is a rich blue coloured oil. It is a very high quality oil with similar therapeutic properties to Roman camomile but also used for stress related conditions, menopause etc. This oil is obtained from eastern Europe. The third oil is Camomile maroc (I) its history is less well known. Therapeutically similar to others. Obtained from North Africa and Spain.*

Carrot seed *(Daucus carota)*
- ☻ Sweet earthy pungent smell. Obtained from seed.
- ▣ Europe, Asia, North Africa. Oil obtained from France.
- ☺ Liver and gall bladder. Tonic effect on the body, skin conditions, excellent for a dry, chapped skin.
- ☯ Strengthens inner visualisation.

Cedarwood *(Cedrus atlantica)*
- ☻ Musky, smoky odour. Distilled and obtained from wood.
- ▣ Atlas mountains in Algeria. Oil from Morocco.
- ☺ Bronchial and urinary conditions e.g. cystitis.
- ☯ Thought to strenghthen spiritual qualities. Wood used to build temples.
- ☹ Not to be used during pregnancy.

The Essential Oils

Citronella *(Cymbopgon nardus)*
- ❀ Fresh lemony odour. Obtained from grass.
- 🗐 Sri Lanka.
- ☺ Stimulating oil. Makes a good insect repellent.
- ☹ Avoid during pregnancy.

Clary sage *(Slavia sclarea)*
- ❀ Sweet, nutty, warm aroma. Obtained from flowers.
- 🗐 Southern Europe. Oil obtained worldwide.
- ☺ Deeply relaxing, Soothes and relieves migraine, asthma, cramps, digestive pain etc. Strengthens the body during convalescence.
- ☹ Not to be taken with alcohol. Not to be used during pregnancy.

Cypress *(Cupressus sempervirens)*
- ❀ Woody smell. Obtained from leaves and cones.
- 🗐 Eastern Mediterranean. Oils from France, Spain, and Morocco.
- ☺ Oversweating, fluid retention, incontinence, painful, heavy menstrual flow.
- ☯ Transition to a new lifestyle, e.g. moving, divorce etc.
- ☹ Not to be used during pregnancy.

Elemi *(Canarium luzonicum)*
- ❀ Fresh, light, lemony, spicy scent. Obtained from tree gum.
- 🗐 Philippines.
- ☺ Stress, inflammation, infectious conditions.
- ☯ Harmonises room atmosphere. Good for group meditations, healing: balances energies.

Eucalyptus *(Eucalyptus globulus)*
- ❀ Refreshing aromatic camphor odour. Obtained from leaves and twigs.
- 🗐 Australia and Tasmania. Obtained from Spain, Brazil, Russia, China, USA.
- ☺ Colds, flu, (antiviral and antibacterial), muscular aches and pains,
- ☯ Purifies room atmosphere e.g. after arguments or rows.
- 📖 One of the most potent antiviral oils in Aromatherapy.
  Various chemotypes exist :
  Eucalyptus lemon (citriodora CT citronnellal). Particularly effective against Staphylococcus bacteria most common in throat infections.
  Eucalyptus peppermint (dives CT piperitone). Similar to Globulus, not so strong.
  Eucalyptus blue gum (globulus). Purifier, colds, flu, antiviral/bacterial,

45

analgesic, muscular.
Eucalyptus Australian *(radiata CT cineole)*. Used when other oils cause skin sensitisation.
☹ Do not use with homeopathic medicine.

Fennel *(Foeniculum vulgare var. dulce)*
✿ Strong aniseed, camphor-like. Obtained from seeds.
▭ Mediterranean. Oil obtained worldwide.
☺ Physically clears toxins e.g. alcohol, 'junk' food, fasting, relieves the digestive system, cellulite, regulates PMT.
☯ Protects from negative energies.
☹ Do not take during pregnancy. Avoid if epileptic.

Frankincense *(Boswellia thurifera or Carteri)*
✿ Lemony, woody, camphor scent. Obtained from tree gum.
▭ Red Sea. Oil obtained from Africa, China, Arabia.
☺ Soothes and relieves respiratory infections, calms coughs; skin care; urinotract infections.
☯ Meditation and connection with the Divine, slows and calms breathing.

Geranium *(Pelargonium graveolens)*
✿ Beautiful, aromatic, fresh, rose-like scent. Obtained from flowers, leaves, and stalks.
▭ South Africa. Oil obtained from Egypt, Russia and China.
☺ Skin healing, balancing, stimulates and balances the adrenal glands. Good for mood swings and stress. Antidepressant. Contains a plant hormone which helps balance the body's hormonal or endocrine systems. Good for regulating the menstrual cycle and relieves PMT.

Ginger *(Zingiber officinale)*
✿ Warm, spicy, aromatic, peppery scent. Obtained from roots.
▭ Asia. Oil obtained from tropical areas.
☺ Soothes arthritis, rheumatism; stimulating, warming; colds, flus.
☹ Slight skin irritant.

Grapefruit *(Citrus paradisi)*
✿ Citrus, tangy, fresh scent. Oil obtained from rind.
▭ Asia. Oil from California.
☺ Skin care, acne, circulation, sore muscles, colds, flu.

Hyssop (*Hyssopus officinalis*)
- ❀ Warm, spicy camphor scent. Obtained from leaves and flowers.
- 🗺 Mediterranean and Asia. Oil obtained from France and Hungary.
- ☺ Respiratory and chest infections, reduces mucus.
- ☹ Avoid during pregnancy, if epileptic or suffering from high blood pressure, NB contains the mildly toxic Pinocamphene.

Jasmine Absolute (*Jasminum officinale var. glandiforum*)
- ❀ Eastern, exotic, floral sweet-scented oil. Obtained from flowers.
- 🗺 China, India, Asia. Oil obtained from India, China, amongst other countries.
- ☺ Luxurious, beautiful, deeply relaxing and nourishing. Good for uterine and menstrual cramps, male sexual impotence, pain relief, and strengthens contractions in childbirth.
- ☯ Unites the feminine and masculine aspects. Sexual problems. Unites with the angelic kingdom.
- ☹ Do not use during pregnancy
- 📖 Jasmine Blend. *Due to the high cost of Jasmine oil, it is usually sold already blended in vegetable oil in a 5% proportion.*

Juniper berry (*Juniperus communis*)
- ❀ Strong, rich, slightly peppery scent. Obtained from berries.
- 🗺 Northern hemisphere. Oil obtained from Europe and Canada.
- ☺ Detoxifies body; cystitis, genital infections, strong antiseptic, acne.
- ☯ Cleanses negative energy.
- ☹ Do not use during pregnancy.

Lavandin (*Lavandula intermedia*)
- ❀ More camphor and woody odour but similar to Lavender. Obtained from flowers.
- 🗺 South France where the oil is also obtained.
- ☺ Similar to Lavender but not so sedative.
- 📖 *True Lavender is cross-pollinated with Spike Lavender to produce Lavendin.*

Lavender (true) (*Lavandula angustifolia*)
- ❀ Beautiful, sweet, aromatic, fruity scent. Obtained from flowers.
- 🗺 Mediterranean. Oil obtained from Europe, Russia, Turkey.
- ☺ Burns/skin healing, colds, coughs, sleeping difficulties, insomnia, headaches, muscular pain, antiseptic, cuts and scratches, all infections, analgesic (gives pain-relief), antibacterial; pregnancy, labour pains.

The Essential Oils

- ❋ Balances and harmonises chakras, moods; relaxing. Is one of the most versatile and popular oils.
- 📖 *Lavender is the most widely used oil due to the fact it has so many diverse qualities and effects. It is an all round healing oil suitable for most conditions. This is because it is a highly complex oil containing over 200 components, each having a different beneficial effect on the body. The body only uses what it needs from the oil.*

Lavender spike (*Lavandula latifolia*)
- ❋ Fresh camphor odour. Obtained from flowers.
- 🗒 Mediterranean. Oil obtained from Europe.
- ☺ Respiratory problems and headaches.
- 📖 *Lavender spike is a much stronger, more camphor-scented oil than Lavender true. For its other properties see Lavender true.*

Lemon (*Citrus limon*)
- ❋ Fruity, refreshing, light citrus scent. Obtained from rind.
- 🗒 Asia. Oil obtained worldwide.
- ☺ Stimulates the white blood corpuscles to strengthen the body's immune system, e.g. very anti-infectious, reduces fevers, stops bleeding, cuts etc. counteracts acid digestion. Bactericide.
- ☹ May cause skin irritation. Phototoxic.

Lemongrass (*Cymbopogon citratus*)
- ❋ Lemony, fresh, light scent. Obtained from grass.
- 🗒 Asia. Oil obtained from Asia, Africa, India.
- ☺ Strengthens the body and is very stimulating. Antiseptic, kills bacteria.
- ☹ Can cause skin irritation in high concentration.

Mandarin (*Citrus reticulata*)
- ❋ Fruity, orange-like, sweet scent. Obtained from rind.
- 🗒 China and Far East. Arrived in Europe in 1805 and in USA 40 years later, renamed as the tangerine. Oil obtained from Europe, USA, Middle East.
- ☺ Digestive problems. Mild and safe, good to use with children.
- ❋ Connects with the inner child, happiness.

Marjoram Sweet (*Origanum marjorana*)
- ❋ Camphor-like, peppery scent. Obtained from flowers.
- 🗒 Mediterranean, North Africa. Oil obtained from Europe, North Africa.
- ☺ Respiratory and infectious conditions, insomnia, warming, gives pain-relief, sedative.

- ☯ Diminishes sexual desire, soothes loneliness.
- ☹ Do not use during pregnancy.

Melissa (Lemon balm) (*Melissa officinalis*)
- ✿ Sweet, lemony, light, pleasant scent. Obtained from flowers and leaves.
- 🗒 Mediterranean. Oil obtained from Europe and Russia.
- ☺ Allergies, relaxing, antiviral.
- ☯ Comforts the dying and bereavement, relieves fears and phobias.
- ☹ Use in low concentration. Possible skin sensitisation.
- 📖 *Note. Melissa is the most commonly adulterated oil due to its very high price.*

Myrrh (*Commiphora myrrha*)
- ✿ Deep, smoky, earthy scent. Obtained from tree gum.
- 🗒 N.E Africa and Asia where oils are still obtained.
- ☺ Heals wounds, antifungal, ulcers, colds, coughs, soar throats, antiseptic, anti-inflammatory.
- ☯ Deepens spiritual connection, clears base chakra blocks, has a grounding effect.
- ☹ Emmenagogic - (can induce or assist menstruation), do not use in pregnancy.

Neroli (Orange Blossom) (*Citrus aurantium var. amara*)
- ✿ Flowery, light, refined, orange-like, very exotic and beautiful scent. Obtained from flowers.
- 🗒 Far East, oil obtained from Italy, North Africa, USA, France.
- ☺ Luxurious and deeply soothing. Uplifts, antiseptic, aphrodisiac, sedative.
- ☯ Reconnects with one's Higher Self (intuitive abilities), helps to clear the crown chakra, antidepressant, good for anxiety, exams etc.
- 📖 *Like Jasmine, Neroli is usually blended in vegetable oil (5%) because of its high cost.*

Niaouli (*Melaleuca viridiflora*)
- ✿ Sweet, fresh, camphor odour. Obtained from leaves and twigs.
- 🗒 Australia where oil is obtained.
- ☺ Antiseptic, e.g. for acne, cuts, and respiratory infections.

Orange (Sweet) (*Citrus sinensis*)
- ✿ Sweet, warm, orange-like scent. Obtained from rind.
- 🗒 China. Obtained from USA, Mediterranean, Brazil, Israel.
- ☺ Aids digestion, diarrhoea, relieves digestive cramps, antidepressant, antiseptic, healing, anti-inflammatory.
- ☯ Brings simple joy.

The Essential Oils

☹ Can cause skin irritation in high concentration.
📖 The Orange tree *(citrus Aurantium v.amara)* produces 3 different essential oils.
 1. Neroli from orange blossom.
 2. Petitgrain from leaves.
 3. Orange oil from rind of fruit.

Palmorosa *(Cymbopogon martinii var. martinii)*
✿ Rosy, geranium-like floral scent. Obtained from grass.
▤ India. Oil obtained from Africa and Brazil.
☺ Skin care, stimulates cellular regeneration, skin infections.

Parsley seed *(Petroselinum sativum)*
✿ Warm, spicy, sweet scent. Obtained from seed.
▤ Mediterranean. Oil obtained from France, Germany, Holland, Hungary.
☺ Releases toxins; arthritis, indigestion.
☹ Avoid during pregnancy. Can be an irritant.

Patchouli *(Pogostemon cablin)*
✿ Sweet, rich, earthy scent. Obtained from dried leaves.
▤ Asia. Oil obtained from China, Asia, S. America.
☺ Skin care, fungal infections such as athlete's foot etc., anti-inflammatory.
☯ Base chakra, grounding to the earth.

Pepper (black) *(Piper nigrum)*
✿ Very strong, pungent, warm, spicy scent. Obtained from pepper berries (corns).
▤ India. Oil obtained from India, Asia, China.
☺ Stiff muscles after exercise. Digestive system, antiseptic, revitalising, very strong stimulant, excellent when tired and needing energy.
☹ Can be a skin irritant.

Peppermint *(Mentha piperita)*
✿ Minty, refreshing scent. Obtained from flowers and leaves.
▤ Propagated from the 17th century in England. Naturalised in Europe and USA. Oil obtained from Europe, Russia, USA, China etc.
☺ Digestive system; soothes, eases cramps, stimulating, warming; colds, flu, headaches.
☯ Inferiority, pride, helps clean moral living. clears the mind. Associated with cleanliness and ethical living.
☹ Can cause skin irritation in high concentration. Avoid during pregnancy. Do not use with homeopathic medicine.

- Combines well with Lavender.

Petitgrain (*Citrus aurantium var. amara*)
- Fresh, floral, citrus scent. Obtained from leaves and twigs.
- China and India. Oil obtained from France and North Africa.
- Uplifting, antiseptic, aphrodisiac.
- Reconnects with the Higher Self, balances the crown chakra, antidepressant, good for anxiety, exams, etc.

Pine needle (*Pinus sylvestris*)
- Strong, refreshing, piny scent. Obtained from pine needles.
- Eurasia. Oil obtained from Europe, Russia.
- Chest infections, colds, sore throats, catarrh, muscular pains. It cleanses the body of infections and toxins and is an expectorant and stimulant.
- Can cause skin irritation in high concentration.

Rose absolute (*Rosa centifolia*)
- The Queen of oils. Deep, sweet, rosy, floral scent. Obtained from rose petals.
- Persia. Oil obtained from Europe, China, North Africa.
- Female reproductive system, regulates menstrual cycle, conception for both male & female, antidepressant, postnatal depression, female sexuality, aphrodisiac.
- Associated with connecting human love with divine love, opens the heart chakra, devotion, soothes grief, connects with the angelic kingdom, strengthens the sacral chakra.

Rosemary (*Rosmarinus officinalis*)
- Fresh, woody, camphor scent. Obtained from leaves and flowers.
- Europe. Oil obtained from France, Spain, and Tunisia.
- Stimulates the central nervous system (CNS), e.g. loss of smell, poor sight, mind-stimulant; MS (multiple sclerosis), respiratory tract conditions, analgesic, muscular pain, antiseptic.
- Psychic protector, clears thoughts.
- Do not use during pregnancy. Do not use if suffering from epilepsy.
- *Various chemotypes are available.*
  1. Rosemary CT borneone - Contains borneone. Good for the respiratory system, muscles, cramp.
  2. Rosemary CT cineole - A good expectorant, anti-infectious.
  3. Rosemary CT verbenon- Mucolytic (breaks down mucus), skin care.

The Essential Oils

Rosewood (*Aniba rosaedora or Ocotea caulata*)
- Sweet, woody, floral scent. Obtained from wood chippings.
- Amazon region. Oil obtained from Brazil and Peru.
- Clears the head, headaches, calms nerves, antibacterial.
- Stimulates and balances the crown chakra; calming, good for meditation.

Sage (*Salvia lavendulaefolia*)
- Strong, camphor, woody scent. Obtained from leaves.
- Spain, from where the oil is obtained.
- Relieves pain, warming, very strong stimulant.
- Promotes wisdom and intuitve abilities, hence its name.
- Toxic due to thujone: safer to use Clary Sage (a milder type of Sage). Do not use during pregnancy.

Sandalwood (*Santalum album*)
- Musky, sweet, woody long-lasting scent. Obtained from wood. Brings the smell of India.
- India and Asia. Oil obtained from Mysore in India.
- Rejuvenates dry skin, urinary conditions, e.g. cystitis. Antiseptic, good for dry coughs.
- Stills mental restlessness. Good for meditation; soothing. Links the base chakra with the crown chakra.

Tangerine see **Mandarin**

Tea-tree (*Melaleuca alternifolia*)
- Fresh, camphor, spicy scent. Obtained from leaves and twigs.
- Australia, from where the oil is obtained.
- A powerful immune system stimulant, colds, flu, cold sores, spots, acne, glandular fever, ME, etc. Anti-infectious (antibacterial/viral/fungal).
- *Tea-tree is one of the most powerful immune system stimulants known to me. It also combines all three anti-infectious qualities: antiviral, antibacterial and antifungal. There has been much research in recent times about this wonderful oil from Australia.*

Thyme (*Thymus vulgaris*)
- Strong, camphor, spicy scent. Obtained from leaves and flowers.
- Spain and Mediterranean. Oil obtained mainly from Spain and some worldwide.
- Colds, flu, mouth/throat and urinary infections; stimulates and

The Essential Oils

- strengthens the mind and body and the immune system; mental concentration, e.g. good for dreamy people, exams.
- ☹ Can cause skin irritation in high concentration. Do not use during pregnancy.
- 📖 *Various chemotypes CT are available*
  THYME CT LINALO- Gentle non-irritant, antifungal ,antiparasitic.
  THYME CT GERANIOL (Grown in high altitude) - Stronger than linalol, good for the female reproductive system, candida.
  THYME CT THUJANOL 4* Very antiviral and anti-pathogenic, stimulates the circulation.
  THYME CT THYMOL* Very strong anti-pathogenic effect and very stimulating (grown in low altitude)
  THYME CT CARVACROL* Very strong anti-pathogenic and very stimulating.
- ☹ *These chemotypes are strong skin irritants.

Vetivert (*Vetiveria zizanoides*)
- ❀ Deep, earthy, smoky, woody scent. Obtained from roots.
- 🗺 India and Sri Lanka. Oil is obtained from Java, Haiti and Reunion.
- ☺ Deeply relaxing, reduces stress, refreshing.

Ylang Ylang (*Cananga odorata genuina*)
- ❀ Very sweet, exotic, floral, strong scent. Obtained from flowers.
- 🗺 Tropical Asia. Oil obtained from Madagascar and Reunion.
- ☺ Heart conditions due to stress, skin care, antidepressant, sedative, aphrodisiac, very calming, aids breathing.
- ☯ Dispels anger, creates a peaceful atmosphere.
- 📖 *The highest quality Ylang Ylang is from the first distillation and is called Ylang Ylang Extra. The second highest quality is Ylang Ylang 111 or the second distillation. The 3rd and 4th distillation are of a much lower quality.*

53

CASE HISTORIES

I have selected these case histories to inspire you and to demonstrate clearly the power of healing that is available through th combination of nature's oils and a belief in our own healing abilities. The names in these accounts have been changed.

MS (MULTIPLE SCLEROSIS)

Anne, aged 62, arrived very exhausted and had difficulty walking. Climbing my stairs was a big obstacle. She was at first suspicious of yet another treatment. For the last three years she had been virtually bedridden and the many different treatments she had tried (including acupuncture, homeopathy, orthodox medicine and osteopathy) had all made her feel worse. Anne had no energy and could be active for only one or two hours a day, but had conserved her available energy in order to get to this treatment. Anne suffered severe muscle-pain, headaches and was unsteady walking. She he had nearly given up any hope of recovery and was forced to accept that she would, in time, steadily deteriorate.

Anne's medical history was complex. She had received many treatments and surgical operations for a variety of complaints including her back and reproductive organs. Her personality was fairly rigid yet she was looking for answers and hope. She easily gave her power away to those who supposedly knew more than she did. I explained that somewhere in her there was great wisdom that knew what her most appropriate treatment was and that in time, with help, she would become her own healer. I would help her with diet, exercises such as yoga, relaxation techniques and with the use of essential oils at home.

First treatment.
I used Rosemary to stimulate the central nervous system, Tea -Tree to act as an immune system stimulant and antiviral agent, and Lavender oil to soothe the pain in her muscles. I gave her exercises to do and suggested a purifying diet and drinking fresh vegetable juicto cleanse her body.

Second treatment 1 week later
Anne reported that she already had more energy and felt hopeful for the first time in years. Hardly believing this new strength, she was frightened of

becoming weaker again. I gave her the same essential oils as in the first treatment to use at home. She had done a lot of yoga exercises and was working very hard and was also developing her intuitive abilities.

Third treatment 2 weeks later

Anne had continued improving at a fast rate to our mutual pleasure and surprise. She was taking longer walks and already planned to see friends for the first time in years. She continued to use the same essential oils at home, to do a lot of yoga and meditation, and to drink fresh vegetable and fruit juices.

Fourth treatment 3 weeks later

Anne arrived looking so much younger and stronger. She was spending most of the day up and about and was planning on going on holiday. I suggested she take things very carefully and not rush into anything although I left the decisions to her. She was very excited and grateful for feeling so much better. The combination of Aromatherapy and Anne's hard work at home with her exercises, diet and meditation had certainly benefitted her.

Anne continued to come for five more treatments and steadily improved to a point where she is living an 80% rather than a 10% normal life.

MYALGIC ENCEPHALOMYELITIS (ME)

Mary, aged 29, was diagnosed with ME two years ago by her doctor. She came to visit me looking vulnerable, tired and pale.

She had very little energy, severe headaches, and such a sensitivity to light and sound that it caused her great pain and emotional suffering. Her heat regulation was disturbed so that she felt alternately very hot and cold. She was able to get up for only about an hour a day and she rested most of the time. Luckily, she had friends and family who were able to help her with the shopping and everyday work. Underlying these physical symptoms were fear, anxiety, doubt as well as a huge feeling of "Am I ever going to get better?". Her symptoms varied from week to week: sometimes she felt stronger, at other times much weaker. Her underlying exhaustion was always there.

Mary had consulted other practitioners besides her own sympathetic, yet unhelpful, GP. She had tried acupuncture for six months, homeopathy for a year, and a healer.

One year before getting ME, Mary had contracted Glandular Fever (Mononucleosis) with which she had been ill for two months, however, prior to that she had suffered no other major illnesses.

Before ME, Mary's diet had been variable: sometimes healthy but often with irregular eating times and often 'junk' food. When she came to see me, her diet had been rapidly changing and was becoming more wholesome and balanced. She avoided meat, chose organic food, some fish, salads, vegetables, fruit and grains. She was also taking vitamins and other dietary supplements but took almost no exercise.

Before being diagnosed with ME, Mary had found her life overwhelming. She had tried to be successful but received no satisfaction from her work or achievements. She felt constantly the need to prove her success in order to be liked.

First treatment.
After taking account of all the above factors, I chose the following oils to start her treatment. Rosemary to strengthen the central nervous system and to help her over-sensitivity to light and sound. Tea Tree for its antibacterial, antiviral, and immune system boosting properties. Lavender for its analgesic properties and because it helps relieve muscle pain, headaches, and is generally soothing.

We then talked about a positive approach to her inner anxieties and illness. I suggested that ME may come to us in order to reharmonise our whole being: that our whole life may have become so out of harmony that our body can no longer tolerate the situation. Perhaps ME provides the opportunity to rebalance our life. With such a point of view, I suggested that we could change our attitude to illness and see it as a helpful friend rather than a disabling enemy which we must destroy at all costs.

Second treatment.
Two weeks later, Mary was still very weak. She had very strong headaches and found it difficult to sleep because of her sensitivity to noise and light. I suggested Frankincense to calm her, to slow her breathing rate and to help her connect to her True Self and intuition, Camomile Roman for general soothing and to help her sleeping patterns, and Tea-Tree to boost her immune system.

Third treatment.
Two weeks later, her condition and symptoms remained unchanged. She was interested in the nature of her illness ("why do you think I need to be ill ") and the special qualities of natural healing and medicine. I suggested various books (see 'Recommended Further Reading'), I used Rosemary to strengthen the central nervous system and to help with her over-sensitivity to light and sound, and continued with the Tea-Tree and Lavender.

Fourth treatment.
Again two weeks later, Mary's condition remained unchanged and she was physically very weak. She wanted to understand more about the spiritual connection in healing and began to show a respect for her illness rather than merely fighting it as an enemy. I told her that the wisest person in her own life could become herself and that she knew better than anyone what was best for her. I recommended more books and discussed the physically and energetically-healing properties of essential oils. I now added Elemi for its balancing healing properties while retaining Tea-Tree.

Fifth treatment.
Now six weeks after the first treatment, there was still no improvement, but Mary, though very weak, had begun to feel spiritually motivated. She expressed a new desire to understand more about her illness. To Elemi and Tea-Tree, I suggested Neroli to help her reconnect to her higher self and intuitive abilities.

Sixth treatment.
For the first time since seeing her, Mary had started to take regular outdoor exercise and gentle stretching movements indoors. Although she found exercise tiring she felt a boost in her energy level. We both felt very excited. I now concentrated on Elemi, Tea-Tree and Frankincense for the above reasons.

Seventh and final treatment.
After a further month, Mary continued improving and her energy levels were higher. She was able to spend up to half of the day active. She now felt a sense of inner purpose and motivation. She recognised that she now had the tools and awareness to enable her to heal herself. We decided this would be a good time to stop the treatment. Mary now felt that she had the confidence, motivation and self-belief to take responsibility for her own health and treatment. I fully supported and encouraged this view and gave her more books to read. I felt she was in safe hands; her self!

ECZEMA

John was 34 years old and held a responsible job. His main reason for coming for treatment was eczema affecting the inside of his knees, elbow joints and, at times, his hands. For the last six months the eczema had been more acute than normal. It had first started about 2 years ago. John's skin was severely cracked and dry in the effected areas and caused discomfort and itching with a resultant irritability and difficulty in sleeping. His condition varied from week to week: sometimes it was very mild, at others quite severe.

He had previously consulted other practitioners: acupuncture for four months one year ago, and his GP two years ago. His GP had prescribed steroids (Tridesilan) for six months which had helped the eczema but induced side effects, and he also needed increasing amounts of steroid cream to achieve the same result. The cream did not actually help the condition itself but merely suppressed its symptoms. As a result, his eczema appeared to be worse after stopping the steroids. Importantly, he did not feel it was right to use steroids.

His medical history was straight forward: he had suffered no major illnesses or injuries and the last time he had been ill was with flu three months before. His diet was a fairly balanced whole food diet with some meat and fish, but sometimes too much chocolate and coffee. He took minimal exercise, such as occasional walks and bike rides.

The main stress in John's life was his work: he had a strong sense of responsibility and was often tired or over stressed at the end of the day. He felt that too much was expected of him and he did not gain enough satisfaction from the work itself. Although he was reserved, he gave the impression of having a balanced personality.

First treatment.
I suggested he use the following diluted oils in an aqueous cream: <u>Benzoin</u> for its anti-allergic properties and <u>Camomile</u> as an anti-inflammatory, to soothe the skin conditions and help stress. I advised John to cut down on stimulants, including chocolate and coffee, and to experiment with cutting out dairy products and wheat and to see a naturopath for advice on diet.

Second treatment.
Two weeks later, John's skin condition was much the same. I recommended that he continued to use <u>Benzoin</u>, <u>Camomile</u> and <u>Lavender</u> and advised him to make up creams of these oils to use at home.

Third treatment.
Two weeks later John's skin had slightly improved. He had changed his diet, the essential oils appeared to help him sleep and he was feeling encouraged. He still felt tired and rundown. I suggested <u>Pine-needle</u> for its antiallergic properties and <u>Melissa</u> for its skin-healing abilities; also to continue with <u>Benzoin</u>.

Fourth treatment.
Two weeks later John's eczema had significantly improved. He felt encouraged by the rapid improvement. I suggested breathing and meditation exercises as an aid to relieve stress at his work. Also yoga to stimulate his circulatory system to help the skin and the whole body. He was to continue with Benzoin and Camomile.

Fifth and final treatment.
The skin condition had made an 80% recovery and no longer caused much irritation or discomfort. We decided to stop the treatment. It had been successful. I advised him to continue using the oils and to respect his stress and anxiety with his work by realising its connection with his eczema.

MEDITATION

There are many types of meditation (see 'Useful Organisations'). The following describes one that has been very helpful to me.

Lie down or sit in a comfortable position, close your eyes and ensure that you will not be disturbed for the next half an hour.

Take 10 or 20 full deep breaths and on each out-breath completely relax the whole body. Then go slowly through the whole body, feeling each body-part in turn, notice any tension and allow it to completely relax. Start with the head (scalp, face, neck) and then proceed to the shoulders, arms, hands, lower and upper back, chest, stomach, lower abdomen, buttocks, genitals, legs, and feet. (Find your own rhythm and the order that suits you.)

When you are feeling completely relaxed, imagine light or energy flowing up the legs and back to the top of the head with each in-breath, while on the out-breath feel this light or energy flow down the front of the body to the feet. Repeat this process for five or ten minutes.

When you have finished, remember all the loved ones in your life and the people you know who are in need; include yourself if appropriate. Send them this sense of relaxation, love, light and healing.

Then slowly open your eyes, get up, and allow any peace or sustenance you have acquired to remain with you.

RECOMMENDED FURTHER READING

BOOKS ON AROMATHERAPY

"A-Z OF AROMATHERAPY" by Patricia Davis
"SUBTLE AROMATHERAPY" by Patricia Davis
both published by CW Daniel Co. Ltd.

"THE FRAGRANT PHARMACY' by V.A Worwood, published by Bantam books

"THE ENCYCLOPAEDIA OF ESSENTIAL OILS" by Julia Lawless, published by Element

"LAVENDER OIL" By Julia Lawless, published by Thorsons/Harper Collins

"TEA TREE' by Julia Lawless, published by Thorsons/Harper Collins

"HOME AROMATHERAPY" by Julia Lawless Thorsons

"AROMATHERAPY AND THE MIND" Julia Lawless, published by Thorsons

"THE NEW HOLISTIC HERBAL" by David Hoffmann, published by Element

"AROMATHERAPY COMMON AILMENTS" by Shirley Price, published by Gaia books

"AROMATHERAPY FOR MOTHER AND BABY" by Allison England, published by Ebury Press

BOOKS ON HEALING AND SPIRITUALITY

"AUTOBIOGRAPHY OF A YOGI" by Paramahansa Yogananda, published by Self Realization Fellowship

"I COME AS A BROTHER" by Bartholomew

"EMMANUEL'S BOOK" ISBN 0-553-34387-4

"OUT ON A LIMB" by Shirley Maclaine

"HANDS OF LIGHT" and "LIGHT EMERGING" by Barbara Brennan

"THE MASSAGE BOOK" by George Downing

"HIDDEN JOURNEY" by Andrew Harvey

"FEEL THE FEAR AND DO IT ANYWAY" by Susan Jeffers

"Your can Heal Your Life" by Louise Hay

"Raw Energy" by Leslie and Susannah Kenton

"Food Combining for Health" by D. Grant and G. Joyce

"Your Inner Physician and You" by Dr. John Upledger

"Self Healing: My Life and Vision" and
"The Hand Book of Self Healing" by Meir Schneider

"Healing into Life and Death" by Stephen Levine

USEFUL ORGANISATIONS

Essential Oil Suppliers

Natural Health Remedies Ltd. (NHR)
10 Bamborough Gdns.
London W12 8QN
0181 743 9485
(High quality organic essential oils, remedies and Aromatherapy supplies. Selection of books also available).

Other Organisations

Aromatherapy Organisations Council AOC
3 Latymer Close
Braybrooke
Market Harborough
Leics. LE16 8LN
01858 434 242
The AOC lists nearly all the Aromatherapy schools and organisations and practitioners in Britain.

BCMA (British Complementary Medicine Association)
9 Soar Lane
Leicester LE3 5DE
Tel. 0116 242 5406
Fax. 0116 242 5496
Lists a huge number of alternative practitioners in all disciplines, schools and organisations in Britain.

Useful Organisations

Meditation Centres

Self Realization Fellowship (SRF)
0171 286 1524 enquiries for Britain
001 213 225 2471 HQ world enquiries
Silent meditation and chanting

The Philosophy School
90 Queen's Gate
London SW7
0171 373 4331
"Ways to Harmonious Living"

Yoga

Iyenga Yoga
Telephone 0171 624 3080
Centres all round Britain

Sivananda Yoga Centre
49 Felsham Road, London SW15
Telephone 0181 781 0160

British Wheel of Yoga
Telephone 01529 306851

Magazines on Healing

"Caduceus"
Telephone 0192 6451897

"Planetary connections"
Telephone 01386 858 694 PO Box 44, Evesham, Worcs, WR12 7YW

"Resurgence"
Telephone 01208 851304

"International Journal of Alternative & Complementary Medicine"
Telephone 01932 874333

GLOSSARY

ANALGESIC - Gives pain relief.

ANTISEPTIC - Destroys or kills microbes (viruses and bacteria).

ANTISPASMODIC - Relaxes and soothes involuntary muscles (e.g. digestive system).

APHRODISIAC - Stimulates sexual desire.

ASTRAL - Heavenly Realm or Subtle universe.

BACTERICIDE - Destroys or kills bacteria.

CHAKRA - Energy centre of the body (or spinal centre). There are seven main chakras: 1. Top of the crown. 2. Middle of the forehead (in between the eyebrows) 3. Throat. 4. Heart or chest. 5. Solar plexus (stomach). 6. Sacral, below the navel (2 inches). 7. Root, at the perineum (in between the anus and the sex organs).

CHEMOTYPE - See under the section 'How Essential Oils are Obtained'

DIURETIC - Stimulates urine excretion.

EMMENAGOGIC - Induces or assists menstruation.

ENDOCRINE SYSTEM - The system of glands in the body which secrete hormones, help fight infections and balances the body's function.

EUPHORIA - A feeling of great elation, especially when exaggerated.

MEDITATION - Deep relaxation and contemplation. Methods vary according to spiritual/religious practise.

PENOCAMPHENE - A chemical component of the Ketone group found in some essential oils, generally has a very strong effect on the body. Often helps the upper respiratory tract.

PHOTOTOXIC - When oils react with the skin in bright sunlight to casue discolouring.

POSTNATAL - After childbirth (PRENATAL - Before childbirth).

SYMPATHETIC NERVOUS SYSTEM - Related to fight and flight response. (e.g. increased heart-rate etc.)

THUJONE - A chemical of the Ketone group found in a few essential oils that are toxic. These essential oils are generally not used in Aromatherapy.

TONIC - Strengthens and enlivens parts or the whole of the body.

TOXINS - Substances or poisons which have a negative or adverse effect on the body's functions.

URINARY or URINO - Relating to the parts of the body that participate in urine excretion - (bladder, urethra, kidneys).

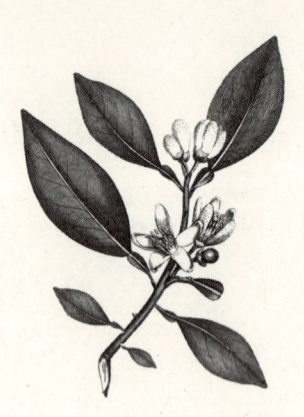

Cover design and Layout by Peter Zinovieff [*]

Electronic typesetting in Pagemaker. Typefaces: Adobe Garamond, Caslon Openface.

Printed on 100% recycled paper.

[*]DPZ GRAPHICS, 1 Cyprus Road, Cambridge, CB1 3QA,
Telephone (44) (0)1223 572780 Facsimile (44) (0)1223 572781 Email petzin@dial.pipex.com